KETO KID

KETO KID

*Helping Your Child
Succeed on the
Ketogenic Diet*

DEBORAH SNYDER, DO

Demos

Demos Medical Publishing, LLC
11 West 42nd Street
New York, New York 10036

Visit our website at www.demosmedpub.com

LIBRARY OF CONGRESS CATALOGING-IN-PUBLICATION DATA
Snyder, Deborah.
   Keto kid : helping your child succeed on the ketogenic diet / Deborah Snyder.
     p.   cm.
   Includes bibliographical references and index.
   ISBN-13: 978-1-932603-29-3 (pbk. : alk. paper)
   ISBN-10: 1-932603-29-8 (pbk. : alk. paper)
   1. Epilepsy in children—Diet therapy—Recipes.   2. Ketogenic diet.
   I. Title.
   RJ496.E6S69   2007
   618.92'8530654—dc22   2006026756

This book offers strategies to parents of children with difficult-to-control seizures for how to succeed on the ketogenic diet. The book is not intended to be an instruction manual or to offer specific medical advice. A book cannot take into account the specific needs of any individual patient. As with any course of treatment for epilepsy, the author and publisher advise parents to discuss the ketogenic diet with their child's physician.

Special discounts on bulk quantities of Demos Medical Publishing books are available to corporations, professional associations, pharmaceutical companies, health care organizations, and other qualifying groups. For details, please contact:

Special Sales Department
Demos Medical Publishing
11 West 42nd Street
New York, NY 10036
Phone: 800-532-8663, 212-683-0072
Fax: 212-683-0118
Email: orderdept@demosmedpub.com

12 13 14 15 5 4

Made in the United States of America by Hamilton Printing.

CONTENTS

PREFACE

MY FAMILY WAS PLUNGED into the world of pediatric epilepsy that fateful day on April 3, 2003, when my 4-year-old son, Bryce, had his first seizure. Within several months, he was having 20-25 seizures daily and was given a grim prognosis. Multiple drugs were tried and failed. Then, on September 1, 2003, he began the ketogenic diet and we experienced the miracle of seizure-free days.

Despite years of training in medical school and then as a practicing family physician, I was overwhelmed by starting the ketogenic diet. I read and re-read every book and article I could get my hands on, and still was unprepared. I vividly recall spending hours at the grocery stores trying to find the right flavoring or the right toothpaste or the right sweetener. I recall feeling alone and unsupported when I called for help in developing a recipe for a ketogenic grilled cheese sandwich and was told to make it on lettuce! How can you melt a third of a stick of butter with a small speck of cheese on a piece of lettuce and pass it off to a 4-year-old as a grilled cheese sandwich?

The ketogenic diet has given me my son back. He has been off the diet for almost a year and a half and counting. He is seizure-free and medication-free. There was not one day that I regretted him being on the diet; there was not one day when I didn't thank God for the diet.

I've learned that the ketogenic diet is an evolution for the entire family; a process, so to speak. There are many physical changes regarding the food, but even more emotional changes that take place. I've included many practical tips for making the diet easier on a daily basis. I've included a recipe section as well as photos of typical meals. I actually had *no* idea of the meal sizes before starting the diet; I never saw a photo of an example meal. When I made my first recipes, it often took four or five tries to get the food to resemble normal kid-food.

It didn't take long for my husband and I to realize that most family and friends just don't "get it," despite their good intentions. We learned that *we* had to shield our son from temptation and advocate for him on a daily basis to ensure the success of the diet. Many people who know our story have asked how we achieved such great success with the ketogenic diet. Throughout this book, you will find examples of the following ten key tips:

1. LIMIT TEMPTATION—The ketogenic diet was not just a change for my son; it was a change for our entire family. We went through the cupboards and discarded all of the chips and bread and candy and other non-ketogenic foods prior to his diet. We no longer left food out on the counter or elsewhere. The refrigerator was off limits to children. When we walked through the grocery store, we tried to skip the candy and cookie aisle, even if it meant walking farther. For holidays, we focused on family instead of food and usually just didn't put snacks out at all. If my husband and I ate chips, we did it after the kids were in bed.

2. SHARE THE SACRIFICE—As a mother, I firmly believed that I needed to experience a little of the diet to truly understand what my son was going through. I recommend this to ev-

ery parent. Of course, going on the ketogenic diet with my son would be medically unsafe. However, I eliminated candy, cookies, and cakes from my diet. When we were at a party and I didn't eat the cookies or cake that he couldn't eat, it helped him know he was not alone. And I gained an understanding of how good chocolate chip cookies look and smell; I shared in the longing for a candy cane at Christmas time or for a malted milk-ball at Easter. For anyone who told me: "He probably doesn't even miss candy anymore," I told them to give up cookies, cake, and candy for two weeks and then come and talk to me.

3. KEEP AN OPEN DIALOGUE—My son and I talked about his diet on a daily basis. When he grew weary, I reminded him that before his diet he was so sick that he couldn't go to school or ride a bike or play outside. I reminded him of how lucky he was to be seizure-free. We talked about how not having candy and not having seizures is better than eating what he wants but being too sick to do anything. When we said our prayers every night, we thanked God for his diet.

4. SIMULATE FAVORITE FOODS—What kid doesn't like hot dogs or cheeseburgers or pizza? The ketogenic diet is restrictive in calories, but that doesn't mean that the foods have to look and taste awful! I just cringe when I hear of kids who have meat and vegetable meals blended together and fed with a spoon because that's the only recipe they were given! I've worked relentlessly to make recipes to simulate kid-friendly food. If the kids at school had pizza, my son had a keto-pizza. If they had a cheeseburger or macaroni-and-cheese, Bryce had his keto-version. I know that it helped him feel included.

5. MAKE IT FUN—We referred to the ketogenic diet as the "magic diet," a phrase coined in *The Ketogenic Diet: A Treatment for Ep-*

ilepsy by John M. Freeman, MD, et al. We explained that the diet was magic because it made Bryce's seizures disappear. Magic implies fun, excitement, mystery, and entertainment...all things that kids can relate to. Additionally, I probably had the biggest stock of holiday cupcake liners, plates, and napkins than anyone I know. I also used various food colorings and toothpicks on a daily basis to make the meals fun and attractive. I focused on decorations for holidays and parties rather than on food.

6. VALIDATE—I often talked to my son about how much "hard work" the diet involves. When we were at the movie theater and the smell of popcorn was intoxicating, I acknowledged that "I know that your diet is hard for you; this is the hard part of your diet." And I also made sure to stress that I know he can do it!

7. GIVE CHOICES—As much as possible, we let my son make choices at mealtimes. We let him choose if he wanted to eat at the kitchen table with us or on the couch in front of the TV by himself. (Prior to his diet, we certainly didn't let him eat alone in front of the TV, but for the duration of his diet we did whatever it took to ensure that meal times were pleasant for him.) We never demanded that he eat a certain meal. Rather, we asked ahead of time what he wanted to have, or gave him two or three choices, and we made what he wanted. When the recipe called for cream, we let him decide if we used the cream for white milk or chocolate milk or pudding. We asked if he wanted the butter separate or mixed in. We ask if he wanted a fork or a spoon to eat it with. These choices empowered my son, and enabled him to "own it." After awhile, he even suggested new recipes for me to calculate.

8. ADVOCATE AND EDUCATE—People generally just don't "get it" with regard to the strictness of the diet and the amount

of sacrifice it demands from our little ones! When we went to a relative's house and there was a cake on the counter, we put it away. We also did whatever we could to allow my son to be included and as normal as possible. This translated into many phone calls and letters on my part. I talked to his teachers ahead of time and asked their support of the diet, and supplied them with a bag of toys to use for a "trade" when a food treat was given that we weren't prepared for. I sent a note out for Halloween explaining the diet and distributed a toy for him to get at trick-or-treat. I gave clear instructions to babysitters and coaches and Sunday school teachers about his diet and his needs. I enlisted their support to help make it a success.

9. PRAISE OFTEN—Daily, I told my son how proud of him I was for not cheating on his diet. I told him how strong he was. I told him what a good boy he was. I told him what a good job he was doing with his diet.

10. SHOW TOUGH LOVE—When he didn't do a good job, I told him as well. And I set punishments…and I enforced them. There was a zero tolerance policy for not finishing his food. In the beginning, we made him eat the fatty parts of the diet first (like the cream and butter), the protein second (the meat, eggs, or cheese) and the carbohydrates third (the fruit and vegetables). If he didn't eat in a reasonable time, we suspended TV privileges or took away favorite toys. When he was hungry and hovered in the kitchen, I made him get out. When he cheated, we made him skip a meal to make a point, even though the cheat was minor and he was still in good ketosis. We did make a strong impression—cheating will not be tolerated!

The ketogenic diet has forever changed our lives for the better. I am hopeful that this book will give families a better understanding of what lies ahead, and help make the diet just a little easier. I will forever remain passionate about the ketogenic diet and its tremendous benefits, and I pray that many, many other children and their families will be able to experience the miracle of seizure-free days.

Deborah Snyder
November 2006

ACKNOWLEDGMENTS

I AM THANKFUL TO GOD. First, for giving me my wonderful son Bryce. Also for providing my family with the strength and ability to succeed on the ketogenic diet. Finally, I thank God for the opportunity to reach out through this book. It is my deepest hope that it will help many other children acheive seizure control.

I would like to thank several other people who have helped me. Thank you to my husband, Jeff, for spending hours and hours editing my book, for being an extraordinary dad, and for being my true partner in life. Thank you to Dr. Shelley Williams, our pediatric neurologist, for providing excellent medical care for Bryce. Thank you to Dr. Elaine Wyllie for your ongoing second opinions whenever needed. Thank you to Dr. John Freeman for dedicating your life to helping children with epilepsy and for your tireless efforts in improving the ketogenic diet. Thank you also for believing in the need for this book, and for helping to make it happen.

KETO KID

CHAPTER 1

*W*EATHERING THE *H*OLIDAYS

*T*he fall and winter months are the most challenging time to be a child on the ketogenic diet. The three big holidays—Thanksgiving, Christmas/Hanukah, and New Year's—all involve elaborate feasts. The holidays themselves are obstacles, but you and your child actually face three full months of challenges. Most cultures tell us to celebrate special occasions with food—marriage, birth, mourning, and especially the holidays. For some, food is an expression of love or a source of comfort. But for keto-kids, food must be nothing more than nourishment for their bodies.

As parents and caregivers, you must provide plenty of love and comfort in a nonfood form. You can do it! My advice to you is to make your number one goal for the holidays to be focusing on family and fun rather than on food. The more planning and preparation you do to be ready, the better you will face the challenges.

In my family, the first major holiday after starting on the ketogenic diet was by far the most daunting for us. With scarcely two months of the diet under our belts, just the idea of making it through was overwhelming for my husband and me. Do we feast on Thanksgiving? Should we invite family? What should we serve? What about the young cousins? The questions came up one after the other. So we planned ahead extensively, and we found that we had a wonderful time! And you can, too! Every holiday and every year will get a little bit easier.

We learned how to prepare meals with several side dishes that Bryce, our son, didn't like. That way, we could still "feast" and it didn't bother him as much. For Christmas one year, I made a roast beef, crab-stuffed oyster shells (well, I bought those frozen!), spinach salad, company potatoes, and corn. Bryce didn't want the roast beef; he had a hot dog and corn. I also found a way to have an appetizer—I set out cold shrimp on the kitchen counter. This was away from the center of activity, and the adults just walked in the kitchen to grab a bite. None of the kids in our family really like shrimp cocktail anyway. The food wasn't staring anyone in the face and it certainly wasn't the focus. For dessert, we had our usual cheesecake. This time, Bryce didn't want his magic cheesecake and so had magic vanilla ice cream with chocolate syrup instead. We waited a few hours after dinner to have our dessert. Everyone was full after dinner, and this allowed me to time the snack to correlate with Bryce's evening snack. For Bryce, the highlights of the day included the presents (of course!) and playing with his three cousins as well as visiting with his family. He easily mastered the concept of focusing on family and fun rather than on food.

You must, as a family unit, learn to focus on family and fun rather than on food. When you really stop to think about it, fellowship is the true purpose of holidays. Gluttony is not. With that in mind, it will be helpful to make small changes in both your holiday traditions and in your expectations.

Let me stress that—*small* changes, such as not setting out a cookie plate. You can and should enjoy your holidays with family and friends. There is no reason why you can't have a wonderful time together, despite the small accommodations you make for your keto-kid.

Living with the ketogenic diet is a process of trial and error. You will learn what works for your child and your family as you go, and you all will improve over time. The key is to plan ahead and to keep an open dialogue with your keto-kid. Be sensitive and validate your child's frustrations. The loss of certain foods (like chocolate and candy canes) is a legitimate loss for your child. There will be a period of "mourning" for these foods as your keto-kid works through his or her feelings. Let your child know that his or her feelings are normal, and that the sadness is legitimate. And remember to end every conversation with a discussion of why they are on the ketogenic diet.

I can't count the number of times that Bryce and I had this discussion. Each time, I listed all the things he couldn't do when he was seizing: ride a bike, go to Chuck E Cheese, go to kindergarten, climb the monkey bars, play without falling on his head, and so on. Then I reminded him that he could do all those things, and more, because of his magic diet. I explained that "it's better to have no candy and no seizures than to be able to eat the candy but have seizures."

Remember: It will get better. You can do it! Every ounce of every sacrifice is worth it!

To illustrate the process, compare my journal entry from our first and second Halloweens:

Halloween, Year 1 (2 months into the ketogenic diet)

I hope Bryce has a fun Halloween! Trick-or-treat is two days away, so tonight I walked around the neighborhood and handed out toys and books from our local dollar store to use as treats. I attached a short note explaining that my 4-year-old is on a special diet and can't have candy or food of any sort. I asked that he be given the treat I left. Mrs. Rossi next door really loves Bryce. Already she gave him a whole bag of treats (she won't be home for trick-or-treat) including a $25 gift certificate to the movie theater. As a teacher she is naturally good with kids, but she's especially good with Bryce. Her heart aches for him as does mine; we both tear up at times when talking about Bryce's epilepsy and his magic diet.

I've been talking to Bryce about getting toys and books for Halloween instead of candy; I thought I prepared him pretty well. Tonight he overheard me on the phone, though, saying he'd be getting toys for treats. He insisted that "toys aren't treats; candy is treats." This began an important conversation between us. Toys can be treats, and the real point of Halloween is dressing up and the fun of going door-to-door. We'll see...this is our first big hurdle, the first holiday on the diet. I did buy Bryce a Wiggles T-shirt and a Berenstain's Bears book that he can have if he "trades in" any candy he gets. We've talked about that also, but seeing as he changed his mind about "treats" (their definition) tonight, who knows how that will go over. I love him so much and so hope that he can focus on the fun part tomorrow....

Bryce is amazing! The night was a huge hit! He loved trick-or-treating for the toys! To give you a visual, he'd walk up to a house and there was a huge bowl of candy that he couldn't have, and tucked somewhere behind it was his treat. He definitely noticed he wasn't getting the candy. He stared at it many times, but he also looked for his treat. I believe Bryce went through an important transition tonight. Once he began to accept his situation, it became easier and easier for him to focus on the fun that he could have. Several of our neighbors (including ones we don't even know) gave Bryce extra gifts that they went out and purchased. Many asked about him and his diet, having never heard of a diet for epilepsy. I cried...but only a little, and they were happy tears. Halloween can be tons of fun on the ketogenic diet! Most of the night was spent smiling and watching Bryce, and holding his baby sister Gracie. Bryce was a dragon and Gracie was a duck! Without his magic diet, I'm sure we would not have gone trick-or-treating; Bryce would have been either too lethargic from the meds or would have been falling on his head due to myoclonic jerks. We are so blessed that his magic diet is working!

Halloween, Year 2 (14 months into the ketogenic diet)

Trick-or-treat in our neighborhood was spectacular! The candy (or rather, lack of) didn't seem to bother Bryce one iota. Whereas last year (two months after starting his diet) Bryce eyed-up the candy as his mouth watered, this year he could care less! I passed out toys and books to about sixty houses this year. As last year, several neighbors gave extra items they purchased themselves. His face lit up with every treat! There were "Wow's" and "Oh boy's" and "Oooohhhh...my favorite." For the houses that didn't read my note (see addendum) and didn't give the toy, we traded in the candy for a Dr. Seuss Leap Pad book. It was a grand trade in Bryce's eyes. There was absolutely no mention of "toys aren't treats," in fact, now the word toy is synonymous with treat! Bryce embraced his special way of trick-or-treating. It was very natural for him this year. He even asked to pass out candy to trick-or-treaters at our door. Picture that: a 5-year-old who can't have candy, having a great time giving it to other children!

At school, there was a carnival put on by the eighth graders—including a haunted house, fortune teller, balloon sculptor, face painter, twister game, etc. There were bowls of candy and toys at each station. The eighth graders who put on the carnival knew about Bryce's diet and included the toys without my prompting; it made me feel wonderful. Bryce, on his own, just picked the toys. I found out ahead of time that there would be a snack of donut holes and juice. I took a cheesecake with orange whipped cream and black chocolate syrup for Bryce to enjoy. He didn't even eat it! He was too preoccupied with playing at the carnival! During his class party, some of his classmates were kind enough to give him a toy as his Halloween treat; for those who gave food, we traded it in when we got home for a big set of Yu-Gi-Oh cards (his favorite!).

As you can see, it really does get easier. And your keto-kid really can have a wonderful holiday, despite the restrictions, if you, the keto-parent (or caregiver) just do a little planning ahead. It can't be stressed enough that every bit of planning and preparation is all worth it!

The tips that follow represent solutions to the challenges we struggled with during the holidays. I hope they make it easier for your keto-kid.

Tips for Weathering the Holidays

🐾 For Halloween, pass out small toys or books to your neighbors (they can be purchased inexpensively at a local dollar store). Distribute them a day or two before trick-or-treating, leaving them in the neighbors' mailboxes. Attach a note explaining briefly that your child is on a special diet and cannot have any candy or food that they are giving out to others. Include a description of your child's costume and ask that they give your special treat instead of theirs.

🐾 There will be parties at school. Talk to your child's teachers, homeroom moms, and principal to find out ahead of time what the treat will be so you can simulate it for your child.

🐾 Send a note home to all of the classroom parents. Ask for advance notice if they plan to send treats to school for any special occasion.

🐾 Supply school teachers with a small bag of inexpensive toys or books to give as a trade in case of surprise treat emergencies.

🐾 Agree with your child about keto-treats ahead of time. Let your child make suggestions and, if possible, use them. Letting your child be involved as much as possible will help your child take ownership of the diet.

🐾 Let your child help choose some of the toys and books. Show him or her the items. This will help build up the anticipation of getting their special nonfood treat.

🐾 If possible, try to be a homeroom mom or at least attend the first few school parties with your child. Be around in case of an unexpected temptation so that you can immediately offer a solution. I once was very glad I took off work to attend Bryce's Christmas party, because one of the primary activities was decorating cookies. Imagine the temptation for a 5-year-old to just lick his icing-covered fingers! He did want to decorate a cookie, so I helped him wash his hands afterwards and was there to remind him that "cookies aren't important." I also offered to trade him the cookie for a Spiderman wristwatch when we got home.

❧ Keep holiday meals simple. There is no reason to go totally overboard with the food. Likewise, you do not have to starve either! Make a nice meal that your family will enjoy, but be mindful to exclude items that your keto-kid previously loved and now cannot have. You can eat those foods in their absence.

❧ I suggest having the first holiday at your home so that you can control the environment. This will not only help your child, but will also help your friends and relatives to see and live the sacrifices your child must make in order to achieve success with the diet. Then, when you do go to a family member's or friend's home (holiday or not), they will have a better understanding of how to create a keto-friendly environment for your child.

❧ Talk with your keto-kid before the holiday about your menu. Choose a few foods that will work for your child as well as for the rest of the family. Make an agreement ahead of time. Ask if certain foods will bother them. For example, my son loved crescent rolls prior to his diet. We then learned that the smells of certain foods really bothered him, so we decided to forego the crescent rolls while he was on the diet.

❧ Be very conscience of smells. In time, your child will forget the tastes of many foods, but the attraction to smells may never go away. The smells of baking cookies, popcorn, toasting bread, and the hot pretzel stand at the mall bothered Bryce for the entire duration of his diet.

❧ We often posted my son's holiday menu on the fridge, and I made him sign his name at the bottom to indicate that he agreed. This kept him from trying to change his mind at the last minute.

❧ Don't serve food "family-style." Rather, keep all the food in the kitchen and have everyone make a plate and bring it into the dining room or to the kitchen table. This helps with the is-sue that your child has a limited amount of food at one sitting, while others can eat endlessly. This tip is particularly helpful for beginners on the diet. After some time, you may be able to transition over to the traditional family-style meals.

🐝 Soon after the meal is over, package up leftovers and get them out of sight. Your child may still be hungry after his or her meal, and seeing an abundance of your leftovers (that he or she can't have) only makes matters worse.

🐝 Consider letting the kids eat first, then go play while the adults eat. This limits the table time for your keto-kid. If you feel that you must all eat together, let your child leave the table as soon as he or she is done. There is nothing helpful about your keto-kid watching you eat.

🐝 The timing of meals is important. If you have an ap-petizer, try to time is so that it coincides with your keto-kid's afternoon snack. Coordinate your dinner time to his or her ap-proximate dinner time. Hold the dessert until his or her snack time. The more you can spread out the food, the more food your child can enjoy.

🐝 Pick an appetizer that your child doesn't like and serve it inconspicuously. For example, we learned to have vegetables and dip and leave it in the kitchen, so the adults could simply go get a bite privately when they wanted. This way, there was no focus on the food and Bryce didn't feel left out.

🐝 We would never have baskets of chips, cookies, or can-dies lying around during the holidays. They weren't necessary and the rest of us could get our fill later. We would forewarn our family and friends that they should fill up on dinner, because the snacking would be limited. My sister would feed her kids "junk foods" in the car on the way to our house, so they would be relatively satisfied when they arrived. Having her children snack before they came helped cut down on snack food requests while they were visiting.

☙ Cheescake is a great ketogenic holiday treat (see the recipe section at the back of the book). For dessert, I would buy a cheesecake for the family, and make a keto-cheesecake for Bryce. I would either match his cheesecake to ours (same blueberry or strawberry topping, nut crust or not, etc.) or I would color his to match the holiday (ex: red cheesecake with green whipped cream for Christmas).

☙ For Thanksgiving, consider making a magic pumpkin pie (see the recipe on page 115). Pumpkin is very low in carbs, so it ends up being a huge serving. In fact, it was so big that it was hard for Bryce to finish, and he asked for a snack-sized pie the next time. Keep the size large if your child is a big eater, or half or quarter the recipe if not.

☙ A lucky few may be able to talk with their team of physicians about giving an extra keto-dessert on rare occasions. This must be something that is ketogenically balanced, such as a half-cheesecake or muffin or one keto-cookie. Not all children can tolerate any extra calories, so you must get permission. Also, this should not be attempted until seizure control is achieved. We were lucky that Bryce could tolerate a few extra ketogenically balanced calories occasionally at special events. We confirmed his tolerance by checking his ketones frequently after the extra food (for him, they always stayed high). If your child's ketones stay high, you know you're minimizing the risk of disrupting ketosis.

☙ Macadamia nuts can be set out as an appetizer for everyone. They are naturally 3:1 so you can calculate a serving for your keto-kid's appetizer also.

☙ Use food coloring creatively. You can make green eggs and ham for St. Patrick's Day, red whipped cream on cheesecake for Christmas, orange and black swirl yogurt for Halloween, and so on.

✲✲ Use fancy paper plates, paper cups, and muffin cups creatively. A macadamia nut snack served in a Halloween muffin cup suddenly becomes a Halloween "treat," and the same old eggs and blueberries for breakfast served on a Santa plate also becomes special. Continue to look for new ways to present keto-foods creatively.

✲✲ Make Jell-O in a holiday color, and use cookie cutters to cut the Jell-O into holiday shapes. Some foods, such as a slice of bologna, can also be cut into shapes and then weighed.

✲✲ Plan a holiday craft to do during the time that you would normally be sitting around snacking and talking. Oriental Trading Co. (www.orientaltrading.com) is a terrific company that is accessible on the Internet. It has hundreds of holiday crafts that you can purchase inexpensively.

✲✲ Likewise, prepare for holidays by doing crafts together (rather than baking cookies or making candy houses, etc.). It can be as simple as a construction paper cutout, or as elaborate as making tree ornaments.

✲✲ Try to save a new dessert recipe to use as a holiday treat. I developed my chocolate chip cookie recipe before Easter and surprised Bryce with the new recipe as his snack on Easter Day.

✲✲ Buy candy molds at a local bakery supply or craft store, along with sucker sticks and colored foils. You can make keto-candy and shape it into various holiday shapes and wrap with appropriately colored wrappers (see the recipe section).

✲✲ Carefully pick and choose holiday events, such as company parties. If the event is filled with non-keto foods as the main focus, it may be better to skip the event rather than trying to get through it...at least at first. A holiday play or a special "family night" showing of Rudolph the Red-Nosed Reindeer (where you can control the food) might be a better idea. We tried to participate in as many social events as possible. However, there were a few times when we stayed home or kept Bryce from school when the event centered around food.

꙳ Sled-riding is an excellent winter holiday activity that is devoid of food. (Although if hot chocolate was previously a favorite, you could make the snack after sled riding include a recipe with cream, and use the cream to make keto-hot choco-late; see the recipe section). If no snack is scheduled, have warm tea sweetened with liquid saccharin.

꙳ Keep up an open and ongoing dialogue with your child about the meaning of each holiday. Talk about the fact that the important part of the holiday is getting together with the people you love and celebrating the special day, not the food. Explain that food is just something that we need to nourish our bodies. It is not the most important thing.

꙳ For Easter, fill plastic eggs with coins and small toys rath-er than with candy. Dollar stores are great for the small toys—we bought bags of plastic bugs and snakes and soldiers and cars, all for a dollar a bag. It does not have to be expensive. Also, Bryce was thrilled to count up his pennies, nickels, dimes, and occa-sional quarters and plan what to buy with them! Bryce's cousins also enjoyed the Easter egg hunt; they were more thrilled with the money and toys than their usual candy treats.

꙳ Remember to call ahead if visiting a friend's or relative's home. Find out what foods will be served, and then prepare a similar meal for your child. Talk with your child in the car about what to expect.

꙳ Explain that the hard part of the magic diet is not being able to eat everything. I personally felt that sharing the sacrifice and refraining from certain unnecessary foods such as cookies and candy was helpful, but others (including my husband) may feel differently. Certainly, you cannot go on the ketogenic diet with your child, but making some small sacrifices will help you to better understand his or her emotions.

🕸 Enlist the help of others. Educate them so they can help advocate for your child. For example, I made sure to explain the limitations of Bryce's diet to my church pastors. They were wonderful about calling ahead when they planned to give a candy or food treat during the children's message so that I could bring an appropriate substitute.

🕸 Consider having a keto-treat kept in the school kitchen to be used as an emergency treat, such as a magic cupcake or magic cookies (see the recipe section). This can be used instead of the regular packed snack if a special treat is given that day by surprise. Of course, it's best to educate teachers and other parents to call you ahead of time if they plan a special snack so you can send in your keto-version!

🕸 Remember that in general, others just don't "get it" with regards to the tremendous sacrifice that maintaining the ketogenic diet takes. Be a shield for your child by doing your best to ensure a keto-friendly environment.

Holidays can and will be wondrous times for you and your keto-kid. Children are resilient and will adapt! You will adapt too! By planning ahead, keeping an open dialogue with your child, validating his or her feelings and, most importantly, by focusing on family and fun rather than on food, your entire family will enjoy each holiday. And you may, just like our family, learn to celebrate the reason for the holiday rather than get wrapped up in commercialism.

There was not one holiday that we regretted being on the ketogenic diet. The diet gave us our son back—and that is more important than any feast! Look at the bright side, with a child on the ketogenic diet, you won't gain those holiday pounds this year!

Every bit of effort is worth it! You can do it!

CHAPTER 2

Coping with the Ketogenic Diet

All the information that my husband and I received about the ketogenic diet from our clinicians was about the physical changes that would take place. We were aware that we would have to weigh all meals on a gram scale, the portions would be small, and they would include very few carbohydrates. We quickly learned, however, that there are just as many emotional changes that take place. The ketogenic diet is a process, an evolution, if you will.

In the beginning, the ketogenic diet was somewhat overwhelming for me (despite my education as a physician with a strong math and science background). I would venture to say that the diet is overwhelming at first for anyone (no matter what their level of education) because of the emotional adjustments that must be made. This is good news, really. You don't have to be smart to have success with the ketogenic diet; you just need to be persistent and keep plugging through! With the passing of each day, the diet became a little bit easier for us to live with and master—and it will for you, too! My husband and I firmly believe that any family can successfully administer the ketogenic diet, if they commit to the diet.

One of the challenges of the ketogenic diet is that the emotional changes occur simultaneously with the physical changes. You must take care to address your child's emotional health as well as physical health. And you must nurture your own emotional health as well. We learned many coping skills along the way. By familiarizing yourself with these skills before your child starts the diet, I hope to make the process easier for you.

Looking back over our two years with the diet, I think that the single most helpful coping mechanism for my son was talking about the diet. It seems so simple to say, but when facing adversity many families don't talk enough. We talked about everything! Before Bryce began the diet, we talked about what would happen during the hospital stay and what changes to his food choices would be made. I bought many new foods for him to try, such as macadamia nuts and blueberries and heavy whipping cream. We discussed his likes and dislikes. I tried a few recipes (guessing at the amounts of each) and let him taste them. This helped reassure him that he'd still get tasty food and helped defray the fear of the unknown. It also helped me get a little practice!

Once the diet began, we talked daily about the sacrifices he was making, how hard it was to be on the diet (validating his frustration), and how proud we were of him for sticking with it! In times of temptation (such as at the movie theater when the smell of popcorn was almost intoxicating) we talked about how not eating popcorn is one of the hard parts of the magic diet and how I know he's a strong boy and can do it, and how lucky we were to be going to the movies because we couldn't do that when he was seizing.

I stressed that it was better to do without candy and treats and not have seizures than it was to eat what he wanted but be too sick with seizures to go out and do fun things. There was a time when Bryce's seizures were at their worst that the only activity he could tolerate was to sit on the couch and watch TV! I often reminded him of this, and together we'd list all of the fun things he could do after his seizures had been controlled with the diet: go to the park, go to the zoo, have play dates with friends, ride a bike, etc. There was not one day that passed that Bryce and I did not talk about his diet. I tried to use every opportunity I could find to validate his feelings and to praise his good choices (to finish "every last drop" and not to cheat). We even role-played at times. For example, we practiced a response to a friend looking at his food and saying "yuck." ("We all have different diets and you don't know if you like it until you try it.")

In addition to talking about his diet, my husband and I employed several other methods to make the diet easier for Bryce. We thought of ourselves as his "shield," protecting him from temptation and doing whatever we could to create a ketogenic-friendly environment.

For example, several days before his diet was initiated, and for the entire duration of his diet, we cleared the countertops of any food. We even took it a step further and cleared our cupboards of many non-keto foods. We did, however, keep a supply of chips and other snacks for us to eat hidden out of sight in the basement. Seeing food sit out on the counter and in the cupboards only strengthens the temptation to try some. Think of what it's like when you go into your kitchen and see a plate of brownies on the counter. You may not have had a thought of eating prior to walking in the kitchen—but as soon as you see the brownies, you want one! You may even get a hunger pain at the sight of the brownies. It's just like that for our keto-kids. But they can't have any extra foods! Simply storing all foods out of sight, and thus out of the way of temptation, can help a lot.

Realize and look for all the ways that you can shield your child. The next step is to proactively look for troubles before they happen, by advocating for your child. My husband and I would call ahead to find out what food would be served at different parties or functions. We would try our best to simulate a keto friendly version for Bryce. However, some parties seemed to focus on food for extended periods of time. We knew that would be trouble! It's much easier for your keto-kid to be strong for short periods of time than for extended periods. Bryce was sometimes a little tired on the ketogenic diet and seemed to wear out quickly. If the only point of the event is food (such as a candy-bar hunt for Easter) you might consider skipping it for a year or two.

Bryce never missed the few events we skipped because we never told him about them! The one exception was when his school had a Thanksgiving Day "feast." It was more like a "food fest." Each mom in his class was to bring in 32 servings of a family recipe. It was clear to my husband and me that there was no way for us to simulate a keto-version of this for Bryce, so we decided to keep him home from school that day. Unfortunately, the school heavily advertised the upcoming day to the students. As a consolation, we arranged for Bryce to have a fun day with his grandmother. He was initially upset but quickly realized that a day with "Grammy" was better than any food!

In addition to advocating, I also engaged in a lot of what I'll call "community education" during the course of Bryce's diet. I invited all of the teachers and staff at Bryce's daycare to a lunch talk about seizures and the ketogenic diet. I provided pizza and pop, as well as handouts which I downloaded from the Epilepsy Foundation website (www.epilepsyfoundation.org).

You don't need to be a doctor to review facts about seizures and the ketogenic diet with others. As a parent or caregiver, you probably know more than any of your child's teachers! If you're uncomfortable speaking in front of others, then consider asking your child's family doctor or pediatrician to help; most will be happy to assist you. I also sent notes to daycare and then to kindergarten regarding the diet in general, as well as the do's and don'ts of the diet (see addendum for examples). I talked to Bryce's friends about the diet, telling them that they could help him by not offering to share their food with him. I enlisted the help of others by having them call me ahead of time if food would be included in an activity, such as at church.

While discussion was the most helpful coping mechanism for Bryce, prayer was the most helpful coping mechanism for me. I relied heavily on my spirituality to get me through each and every day. When I look back at myself over the two years, I see that God carried me many times. Whether you believe in God, Buddha, Muhammed, or some other spiritual force, my best advice to you is to rely on it.

Unfortunately, there will be few people who will really understand what you're going through. Few people really "get it." Even many family and close friends, although they have the best of intentions, will never understand the sacrifice that the diet demands. We had several family members that, despite explaining the diet in detail to them, later asked questions such as, "You mean he can't just have one little bite of chocolate?"

You must foster your own inner strength to help you through the everyday challenges of the diet. Of course, things such as eating healthy foods, exercise, journaling, and a good daily dose of laughter also help. What replenishes your spirit? Have you ever thought about it? If you don't already know, you must learn what restores your sense of well-being and take the time to nurture it! You must try to stay grounded and focused. Take time to recharge and your entire family will benefit.

My husband and I made it a point to periodically go out on our own. Eating out at restaurants was always a special treat. Good food never tasted as good as when we only ate out occasionally. It was easy for a babysitter to give Bryce his snack (which we had already prepared and measured) to allow us a few hours away from the house (and the diet and the seizures) from time to time. The adult time that my husband and I spent together was an important part of coping and recharging for us. When Bryce was at his worst, having multiple daily seizures and declining developmentally, I thought of couples I had known or heard of who divorced because of tragedy in their lives. I wondered if it would happen to us. I remember sharing that thought with my husband, who quickly retorted that our circumstance could also make us stronger. And they have! The reason I believe that we weathered the storm so well is that we communicated and supported each other, and still took time to focus on our relationship.

Whether it be by talking to your keto-kid, advocating, praying, or taking time to replenish your spirit, please do not forget to acknowledge the emotional changes that the ketogenic diet brings! I hope that the following tips will help to make it a little easier on you.

Tips for Coping with the Ketogenic Diet

☙ In the beginning of the diet, try to eat meals similar to your keto-kid so your child doesn't experience such a drastic change. For example, if your child is having a hamburger and carrots, you can have a hamburger, carrots, and a salad (with more meat and vegetables and less butter, of course). Try to include other side dishes for you to eat that your keto-kid does not like.

☙ Do not eat foods in front of your keto-kid that he or she cannot have at all. There is plenty of private time when you can eat candy or cookies if you like. If there are siblings in the house, make it a rule that they must eat such non-keto snacks out of view of your keto-kid.

☙ Create mini-hurdles in your mind (and perhaps on your calendar) to help get through the two years on the diet. For me, the beginning of each month was a mini-victory; one month closer to the end. Looking back, the time went quickly.

🐾 Make a graph of the number of seizures your child had before the ketogenic diet and then the first several months on the diet. It was encouraging for us to see that Bryce was having over 300 seizures per month before the diet, then 150 in the first month on the diet, then 5 the second month, and then none thereafter.

🐾 If your doctor does not "believe" in the ketogenic diet or is not comfortable supervising it, get a second opinion. Two good resources to find a keto-friendly neurologist are Johns Hopkins Hospital and the Yahoo support group website (yahoogroups-ketogenic.com).

🐾 I firmly believe that starting the diet early in the course of uncontrolled epilepsy may play a part in promoting success on the diet. After your child has failed three medications, the chances that the fourth will work are slim. Consider starting the ketogenic diet as early after diagnosis as possible.

🐾 Ask your physician if a prescription for Diastat might be appropriate for your child. It is a rectal valium that can be administered by the parents or caregivers at home in case of a prolonged seizure. We carried it with us for the entire two years on the diet, and then for six months after. It was relieving to know we had it in case we needed it.

🐾 Reward your child with a trip to a dollar store or with a small, inexpensive toy after getting blood work (as well as instead of food treats for special occasions).

🐾 If your child is aggressive because of medications (meds are often continued initially on the ketogenic diet), buy a toy blow-up punching bag for your child to release the negative energy.

🐾 Try to keep things in perspective. As parents, we were

devastated after Bryce had his first seizure. Months later when he was having up to 25 seizures a day, we would have gladly gone back to the former state. Do your best to keep a "glass half-full" approach. It can always be worse!

☙ Pace yourself. One of the best pieces of advice I received was that living with uncontrolled epilepsy (and the ketogenic diet) is a marathon, not a sprint. Know that you're in it for the long haul and don't pressure yourself to do too much at once.

☙ Tivo your child's favorite TV shows so that you can fast forward through commercials. It's amazing how many food and candy commercials are stuffed between cartoon segments!

☙ Barter with your child regarding meals when you have to. For example, if they are demanding magic bacon-and-apple pie and you're out of apples, make a deal that they can have it for dinner the next two days if they eat something else now.

☙ For most young kids, the biggest thrill of the fast food restaurant is getting the toy they see on TV. Purchase a toy for your child when you go to fast food restaurants, even if you're just going through the drive-through for coffee. Most McDonald's let you purchase the toy for a dollar (without the meal). Our local Burger King required paying the price of the entire kid's meal just to get the toy (which we often did).

☙ When eating in, don't serve food family-style. Make a plate for everyone and leave the rest in the kitchen/on the stove. Seeing loads of extra food that is not allowed only makes a hungry kid hungrier! Clean-up will be much easier for you, too.

☙ "Stop and smell the roses," literally. Plan a trip to a botanical garden or the zoo or even just to your local playground. Take time to unwind and relax.

☙ After your child has been on the ketogenic diet a month or two, challenge yourself to take a few steps toward normalcy.

Try going out to a restaurant with your keto-kid. It helps if your child gets to choose the restaurant. Pack a keto-meal in a container and bring it along. Be mindful of what you order (ex: we would never order French fries in front of Bryce because this was a former favorite). Eventually, you have to take the plunge!

🐝 When eating out, have the waitress clear the leftover food away from the table (or place it in take-home containers) as soon as possible. Again, there is no good that can come from your keto-kid seeing your leftovers when he or she may still be hungry and can't have more.

🐝 Remember to call ahead when eating out. There are a few restaurants that actually don't have a microwave or will be unwilling to let you heat a meal in their microwave. Avoid those restaurants, or simply pack something that doesn't require reheating.

🐝 Teach your child helpful phrases such as, "My diet is worth it."

🐝 Praise your keto-kid daily. Simple compliments such as, "I'm so proud of you," and, "You're doing a great job on your magic diet," go a long way toward empowering your child.

🐝 On sick days, offer keto-treats as meals. Our favorites were magic muffins and magic cupcakes (see the recipe section). Each bite is ketogenically balanced, so if you child vomits and loses some or just refuses to finish it, there should not be a problem. These types of food went down better for Bryce than the cream-based eggnog.

🐝 While sick, it is fine to let your child skip a meal or two if your child is unable to eat or hold anything down. Remember to push fluids, however, like ketogenic Kool-Aid or even keto-Popsicles. If your child's illness is severe or lasts longer than a day, always call your doctor.

🐝 Let your child get up from the table and go play as soon

as he or she is finished with a meal. Do not make your child wait until others are done.

🙦 Make whatever reasonable accommodations you have to in order to make mealtimes pleasant for your child. Prior to and after his diet, we required Bryce to sit at the table with the rest of the family for meals. On his diet, we let him eat alone in front of the TV whenever he preferred.

🙦 Especially in the beginning, have your child eat the fat in the meal first, then the protein, and finally the carbohydrate. The fat is the hardest part to eat, usually, but the most crucial in maintaining ketosis.

🙦 At times you will need to exercise "tough love." If our son refused to finish a meal, we'd threaten him with having to skip the next meal. When he was in the kitchen while I was cooking and he whined for "just one bite," I made him leave. When he cheated once with taking a tiny bite of salami out of the fridge, I made him skip the next meal as punishment then we made a sign for the fridge saying "Nobody Allowed in Here Unless They Are a Grown-Up." Because salami is all protein and fat, I knew it wouldn't disrupt his ketosis, but I wanted to make a point: Cheating will not be tolerated! He never cheated again.

🙦 Invite babysitters over for an hour or so to learn the routine while you are home. Let them watch you measure a meal so they can see how exact it all must be. It would be better for you to prepare all foods ahead of time so all they need to do is just heat it up. Show the babysitter how to scrape the container with a spatula, and how to encourage your keto-kid to eat every last drop. Explain what to do if a piece of food falls on the floor (pick it up, clean it off, and give it back to your keto-kid to eat).

🙦 For family birthdays, consider serving cupcakes, muffins, or cheesecake. Your child can have his or her own keto-version (see the recipe section) and you can decorate it to match the rest. This will help your child fit in.

🐝 Instead of treats at school for your child's birthday, take in a helium balloon for every child. Seeing a bunch of 15–20 balloons makes quite an impression on little ones. It will make more of an impact than any food!

🐝 Be careful not to spoil your keto-kid too much. When our son was seizing frequently and when he first began the diet, my husband and I, as well as our family and friends, showered him with small gifts to encourage him. After a few months (when he was well again), he came to expect gifts every time we came home from work and every time people visited. It was harder to undo than it was to do.

🐝 Likewise, remember to continue to discipline your keto-kid just as you did before he or she began to seize. If you don't treat your child like a normal kid, you'll create a monster.

🐝 Buy your child a play kitchen and/or play food. It will help your child work through feelings of mourning for the foods that can no longer be consumed, because your child can pretend to eat whatever he or she wants!

🐝 Be careful to limit smells. For my son, the smells of foods he could not have bothered him the most. There are small steps you can take to help. For example, if we passed by a cookie stand at the mall I would tell Bryce to hold his nose. I also refrained from buying any candles for my house that smelled like food.

🐝 Supervise the first few outings with your child, such as the first day at preschool or the first lunch at school. Explain your child's needs to the teachers/supervisors and provide them with written information they can refer to (see examples in the Appendix). Stand back and observe, and be available for questions. The time you spend this way will be well worth it. The teachers will be more comfortable with your child's needs, and you will be comfortable knowing that the teachers are competent to assist with the diet when you're not there.

🐝 Consider sharing some part of your child's sacrifice.

While it would be medically unsafe for you to be on the diet, too, a little sacrifice on your part will enhance your understanding of what your child is going through. For example, resolve to give up candy or cookies or cakes with your child. I gave it all up; my husband didn't, although his intake of sweets was greatly diminished. For me, it helped me to feel some of what Bryce was feeling, especially during holidays and special events when the sweets were everywhere! I think it helped Bryce too, knowing that he wasn't going it entirely alone. If elimination of all sweets is too much for you to tackle, pick one thing to sacrifice with your child.

 ❧ Ask close friends to discourage their children from snacking during play dates, when possible. My good friends were happy to help; acquaintances generally avoided get-togethers with us (which was fine with me, all things considered). While you cannot expect others to be on the diet also, the people who care about you will gladly make small accommodations to ensure a temptation-free environment for your child. My friends usually took their kids to a fast-food restaurant before coming over for a play date; that way they were full and food was not an issue.

 ❧ At mealtimes, talk with your keto-kid about the fact that "everyone has different diets." I can recall many occasions when Bryce ate his keto-food, his baby sister Gracie ate her baby food, and my husband Jeff and I ate our food. Keeping an open dialogue and openly talking about our differences in a matter-of-fact demeanor helped. Bryce was content with us all having different meals.

 ❧ When it's time to increase your child's calories, ask your dietician if you can increase the calories by the amount of calories in one snack, rather than by the standard 100 calories. Bryce's snack turned out to be 125 calories. We added an afternoon snack and later doubled his evening snack rather than having to add 100 calories and recalculate all of the recipes each time. This will allow you to build on the recipes you already have rather than completely discarding your current recipe book and starting all over.

🕸 Keep in mind that you may be able to be flexible with your child's daily calorie allotment. I never consulted our dietician regarding this, but intuitively it makes sense. At the start of the diet, your child is determined to require x calories. The parents then choose whether to give three meals, three meals and one snack, or three meals and two snacks. The calories are divided accordingly. Thus, I conclude that as long as the meals are ketogenically balanced, it does not matter if more calories (within reason) are given at one meal or not. For example, if you are planning to go to a party in the late afternoon, why not give a snack at lunch time and then let your keto-kid have a lunch and a dinner at dinner time. This will provide plenty of food for your child and prevent him or her from getting hungry during the party (when the temptation for many non-keto foods abounds).

🕸 Try Tom's of Maine Silly Strawberry Toothpaste. When I called the company to get the values, they couldn't quote them to me, but I was told there are natural fruit extracts in the toothpaste. Bryce did fine with it, as long as he didn't swallow it. If he did swallow, his ketones dropped a little. He absolutely hated the other keto-toothpastes, however, because they were all mint-based. The crying and carrying-on over tooth brushing was replaced by giggles when we switched to the Silly Strawberry!

🕸 Be tolerant and try to avoid things that bother your keto-kid. I was shocked to find that 1-½ years into his diet, Bryce was very upset by his baby sister getting to eat a whole cracker. It wasn't that she was eating a cracker (he accepted that we all have different diets); Bryce was bothered that she got a whole piece (it had about a two-inch diameter). On the rare occasions that Bryce had a snack of crackers, we broke them into small pieces to make them look like more or they already were small (like Baby Goldfish crackers). By simply breaking up his sister's cracker into small pieces, Bryce was pacified.

🐟 Role play difficult situations with your child. Before his first visit to a friend's house by himself, we practiced saying, "No, thank you, that's not on my magic diet" if offered a snack other than the one I had packed for him.

🐟 When you have your overnight EEG, ask the technician if he or she will put the wire leads (that attach to your child's scalp) on in your child's room. It was only during our third overnight EEG that this was offered and it made the whole experience much better! Bryce was able to watch TV while the leads were placed, which was an enormous distraction. Compared to the tiny room where we previously had the leads placed, there was plenty of space for me to sit next to Bryce and snuggle, which was a great comfort for him.

With the passing of each day, the ketogenic diet will get easier for you and your child. You will both learn to cope and to adapt. Soon, the ketogenic diet will become a normal, accepted way of life for you. Always be mindful of the emotional changes that accompany the physical changes of the diet. Make sure to include plenty of fun and relaxation in the daily routine for your keto-kid, you as the caregiver, and the rest of your family. Keep an open dialogue with your keto-kid to help your child navigate the daily challenges of the diet. And remember to nurture your own spirit, too, so that you will remain mentally strong throughout the duration of the diet.

You can do it!

CHAPTER 3

KETOGENIC COOKING

Ketogenic cooking is just as much of an art as a science. There is a tremendous learning curve. Recipes that take an hour to calculate and prepare in the beginning take half or a quarter of that time later on. On average, you will spend about two hours per day on ketogenic meal preparation.

I learned many time-saving tricks over the two years that we were on the ketogenic diet, the most helpful being mass production. If you are already making one meal for your child, why not increase the recipe by five or six times and make several meals to freeze for later use? It may take a few extra minutes, but in the long run the "freezer foods" are a tremendous help both when time is short and when the unexpected happens, such as a major spill or if your scale breaks. Freezer foods also enable you to provide choices for your keto-kid.

At the heart of ketogenic cooking is creating recipes that your child will like. Let me say that another way: Success on the ketogenic diet hinges on your ability to provide foods that your child will eat. I can recall hearing stories about kids who were given meals of meat and vegetables all blended together in a food processor. Yuck! If your child is tube-fed, this might work. If not, chances are it will not go over so well.

One of my most frustrating experiences was when I called for help in creating a ketogenic grilled cheese sandwich. Bryce had been on the diet for six months, and really missed his previous favorite meal. It was suggested that I simply substitute lettuce for the bread. How in the heck can I melt a third of a stick of butter and a tiny cube of cheese between two pieces of lettuce and pass it off to a 4-year-old as a grilled cheese sandwich? I was both furious and frustrated, feeling completely overwhelmed that I had little help or support. Luckily, after hours and hours of reading bread labels in the grocery stores to find a truly low-carb bread, my wonderful husband, dad-extraordinaire, located one that worked! That bread discovery quickly led to one of my son's favorite meals—the magic grilled cheese sandwich. I think it made him feel normal.

Let's face it—kids like to eat kid's foods! You will find over one-hundred recipes in Chapter 4, "Ketogenic Recipes," starting on page 43 (including one for a delicious ketogenic grilled cheese sandwich) that are excellent examples of kid-friendly foods.

In this chapter, you will find many tips for making food preparation easier. Remember, it does get easier.

Tips for Ketogenic Cooking

❧ I highly recommend learning to calculate meals yourself. Learning the math was challenging at first, but with practice it became easier and easier. In the beginning it took us 30 minutes or more to calculate meals. In the end, it took 5 minutes or less. Having the ability to calculate meals gives you and your child tremendous flexibility on the diet. It also allows you to let your child be active in meal planning and recipe creation, which helps your child take ownership of the diet and helps promotes success. By recalculating a standard recipe for hamburger and strawberries, for example, you can change the strawberries to include any seasonal fruit or vegetable. Now one meal recipe sprouts into twenty recipes!

❧ In general, measure all meats and vegetables after cooking them. Make sure to pat them dry first. Eggs are one exception—eggs are always measured raw.

❧ Cream is an integral part of the ketogenic diet and has many uses. You can empower your keto-kid by giving him or her choices about how to prepare the cream in the recipes. Changing the cream consistency also adds variety. The many uses of cream are:

❧ White milk—add a few ounces of water and a few drops of liquid sweetener if desired; it's also good without the sweetener.

❧ Chocolate or strawberry milk—add a few ounces of water and a few drops of liquid sweetener, as well as a pinch of sugar-free Jell-O pudding mix, chocolate or strawberry. If your child is seizure-free on the diet, you can substitute a small teaspoon full of Walden Farm's Chocolate Syrup for the chocolate Jell-O.

❧ Hot chocolate—add a few ounces of water and a few drops of liquid sweetener, as well as a pinch of sugar-free chocolate Jell-O pudding mix. If your child is seizure-free on the diet, you can substitute a small teaspoonful of Walden Farm's Chocolate Syrup for the chocolate Jell-O. Heat in the microwave for 30 seconds or until warm.

❧ Whipped cream—add a few drops of liquid sweetener and whip, then use it on top of fruit, cupcakes, or apple pie.

꙾ Pudding—add a few drops of liquid sweetener and a pinch of sugar free Jell-O pudding mix, chocolate or strawberry or any other flavor, and whip. The Bickford flavors can also be used instead of the Jell-O.

꙾ Milkshake—add a few ounces of water, a few drops of liquid sweetener, and a pinch of sugar-free Jell-O pudding mix, chocolate or strawberry or any other flavor, and whip. The Bickford flavors can also be used instead of the Jell-O.

꙾ Smoothie—add a few ounces of water, a few drops of liquid sweetener, and the fruit from the recipe (strawberries and blueberries work very well), and whip.

꙾ Ice cream—add a few ounces of water, a few drops of liquid sweetener, and a pinch of sugar-free Jell-O pudding mix, chocolate or strawberry or any other flavor, and whip. The Bickford flavors can also be used instead of the Jell-O. Then freeze for at least 40 minutes, although you can prepare this days ahead of time. You may also choose to top with two crushed macadamia nuts prior to serving. We called this "sprinkles" and used the macadamia nuts as the free food for the day.

꙾ Cream soda—mix the cream with a few ounces of sugar-free soda.

꙾ Creamsicle—mix the cream with a small amount of sugar-free soda or keto-Kool-Aid and freeze into popsicles. You must take care to measure the exact amount of cream into each popsicle tray and ensure that your child eats all of the popsicle without letting it drip all over.

🐝 Be careful with food values. The protein and carbohydrate values can vary between two different brands of frozen vegetables, or between fresh and frozen vegetables. (Your child will generally get a larger serving with frozen vegetables.) The recipe section in this book contains the brands we found with the lowest carbohydrates. If you find similar foods with lower values, use them because your child will get a larger serving that way.

🐝 There seems to be a "rate-limiting step" to keto-cooking. You will often run out of one critical ingredient. We came to accept late-night trips to the grocery store. You can try to buy certain ingredients in mass quantities, such as macadamia nuts, butter, Irene's gluten bread (stored frozen), canola oil, and Hunt's tomato sauce. It's simply not possible or financially practical to keep on hand a large supply of perishable staples such as cream, eggs, blueberries, and strawberries.

🐝 Try to incorporate your child's meal into the family meal. For example, if you and your keto-kid agree on a hamburger and corn for dinner, make hamburgers and corn for the rest of the family. We would often add a side dish for my husband and myself that Bryce didn't like, such as salad or rice.

🐝 Cook in bulk, as much as possible. Using the above example, you can have one skillet going with a hamburger for your keto-kid (for the current meal and several freezer meals) and one skillet going with seasoned, regular hamburgers for the rest of the family. Steam a large bag of corn. Weigh your child's portion at mealtime, have everyone eat, then after dinner spend an extra 20 minutes measuring the portions for the freezer. Label the lids with permanent marker on masking tape. Be careful to clearly mark if the meal is complete or if cream needs added: "serve with 20 grams of cream."

🐝 Block off time to cook uninterrupted. It is much easier to do mass production cooking when you have no distractions.

🐝 The fat is the most important component of the ketogenic diet, and the part that sticks to the sides of containers! No matter how well you scrape, some of the fat remains. We decided to add about an extra 0.5–1 gram fat (butter, cream, or oil) to the meals to account for the fat that sticks. This definitely improved Bryce's ketosis.

🙊 Use the same bowl to measure multiple ingredients. This prevents losing some of the quantity due to sticking. As above, the part that usually sticks is the fat. This tip would not be for beginners, as there is definitely a learning curve to weighing ingredients on the scale (if you make a mistake, you'll have to throw everything away and start over). After comfort is achieved, however, this tip saves time and keeps the recipe more ketogenic.

🙊 Remember to spray Pam Nonstick Cooking Spray on anything that may stick before baking. You don't have to calculate the Pam into your recipe, and if your meal sticks or burns then you may have to throw it away and start over.

🙊 Most frozen vegetables have lower carbohydrate values than fresh vegetables. Your child will get a bigger portion if you use the frozen vegetables. Also keep in mind that the carbohydrate values differ from brand to brand, so read the labels at your local grocery store for the lowest-carb brand for the vegetables your child will be eating and stick to that brand.

🙊 Many of my recipes call for ground macadamia nuts. I used them as my "flour" and kept a jar full of ground nuts in the fridge at all times. The best way I found to grind the nuts was to put a small handful of nuts at a time in the blender, using a spoon to pull them out and transfer them into a jar.

🙊 Walden Farms manufactures several wonderful products that I was able to use sparingly (1 small teaspoon once or twice daily). These include a Chocolate Syrup, Ketchup, and Maple Syrup. They also make a Ranch Dressing and Barbecue Sauce. These products taste great and really are a treat. They spice up many foods. As they are processed, you should not use when starting the diet (you can use sugar-free Jell-O gelatin and pudding mixes or Bickford flavorings instead). When using the Walden Farm's products, carefully monitor your child's ketosis to assure your child can tolerate these. For 2 tablespoons of Walden Farm's products, there is no protein, fat, or carbs, and no calories. I bought them at Muscarella's Vitamin Center, 3581 East State Street, Hermitage, PA 16148 (724-981-1137). There is also a manufacturer website (waldenfarms.com).

🐾 Bickford Flavors are wonderful and can be used instead of vanilla to add variety to recipes. Use only 5 drops or less per meal. The fruit flavors have natural fruit extracts and so your child may or may not tolerate them (ex: apple and strawberry). The chocolate flavor is great for "magic chocolate milk"; the caramel and butterscotch also taste great. They can be ordered at 216-531-6006 or www.bickfordflavors.com. A 1-oz. bottle is roughly $2.50.

🐾 We found a brand of bread that will work on the ketogenic diet: Irene's Healthy Bakery Gluten Bread. It is stored frozen. For each slice (25 g) there are 3 grams protein, 0 grams fat, and 4 grams carbs. We were able to make our son half of a grilled cheese sandwich with it (1,100 cal/d diet). We learned to cut off the crust in order to achieve a larger sandwich size. We also chose thin slices for Bryce (the slice sizes in each package vary). Irene's Healthy Bakery Gluten Bread comes in several flavors such as white, garlic, and rye. It did lower the ketosis in our son a little (but we still used it). Check your child's ketones after serving to see if he/she can tolerate it. The bakery address is 11462 Nicholson Road, Garrettsville, OH 44231. We got our bread at Muscarella's. Diane was a wonderful help; she would be happy to arrange to ship the bread to you. We also purchased supplements such as selenium from Muscarella's as needed.

🐾 Drinks are one of the easier challenges on the ketogenic diet. Be sure that drinks don't contain hidden sugars such as maltodextrin. Kool-Aid flavors (without maltodextrin) include: Lemon-Lime, Tropical Punch, Cherry, Black Cherry, Blastin' Berry Cherry, and Changin' Cherry Magic Twist. Check the store for new Kool-Aid flavors periodically. I found a new one without maltodextrin several times over the course of our two years on the diet. All of the Wylers flavors have maltrodextrin and therefore cannot be used. Most keto-kids can tolerate small amounts of aspartame (such as found in diet pop); limit drinks with aspartame to 8 ounces per day. Crystal Light Raspberry Lemonade worked well for us; it has aspartame.

🐾 Calcimix is sold over-the-counter, but it is not found on the store shelves; it must be ordered in by the pharmacist. I often used Calcimix to "fortify" recipes with extra calcium, especially dishes like magic waffles, magic macaroni-and-cheese, magic cupcakes, and cheesecake. I occasionally slipped in the extra calcium in addition to the daily calcium supplement because the diet is deficient in calcium.

🐾 I found Cal-Mag-Zinc II to be a much better calcium supplement than the Calcimix. Cal-Mag-Zinc II is in liquid form so it mixes into meals more easily, especially in the cream. Calcimix is a powder and creates clumps when mixed in cream, especially if it's prepared ahead of time. Cal-Mag-Zinc II also has several extra vitamins and minerals, which is always a plus. Its keto-friendly. Cal-Mag-Zinc II can be purchased from Whole Life Nutritional Supplements, 13340 Saticoy Street, Unit B, North Hollywood, CA 91605. Their phone numbers are 818-255-5357 or 800-748-5841. One bottle is roughly $10 and lasts about a month.

🐾 Sugar-Free One-A-Day Kids Bugs Bunny vitamins are available at Target stores. There is also a new Sugar-Free One-A-Day Justice League vitamin.

🐾 Giant Eagle supermarket has Food Club Liquid Sweetener, which is okay for the ketogenic diet. You need the liquid saccharin, not the packets.

🐾 Frothers for cappuccino work great for mixing the small amounts you need to work with. We use frothers to whip cream for "pudding" and "ice cream" as well as to scramble eggs.

🐾 If your child has trouble with bacon (a processed food), you can ask a butcher to thinly slice side pork. It's unprocessed and is what they use to make bacon. It tastes like unsalted bacon and looks just like bacon. We used side pork exclusively, and had our local butcher prepare ten to twenty 1-lb packages of side pork, wrapped individually for the deep freezer. We simply placed a package in the refrigerator to thaw when needed. Our butcher was Lee Hanson at Hanson's Freezer Meats, 247 McClure Avenue, Sharon, PA 16146 (724-981-1950). He was always very helpful and concerned and would be happy to work out an arrangement with you for orders.

🐾 The following websites were very helpful:

🌾 http://health.groups.yahoo.com/group/ketogenic/

This is a support group for parents of kids on the ketogenic diet. There is often sharing of recipes or cooking tips, as well as coping tips. It is excellent.

🌾 http://www.lpch.org/DiseaseHealthInfo/HealthLibrary/
neuro/seizep.htttml

This is mainly an informational site.

🌾 http://www.ars.usda.gov/Services/docs.htm?docid=8964

This is the USDA website for food labels and lists the serving size, protein, fat, and carbohydrate values for all USDA foods. It is very helpful in calculating recipes, especially for things such as meats, fruits, and vegetables that are not always packaged with food labels.

📚 Label all of your freezer food containers using masking tape and a permanent magic marker. Make sure to include the ratio (in case it changes later), the name of the meal, and whether it is complete or needs to be served with cream (ex: write "add 20 grams cream").

📚 Ketogenic mashed potatoes can be made as a rare treat (because they take up a lot of carbs) by mixing 10 grams of potatoes with equal parts of cream and butter. Just mash and serve. They are a thinner consistency than traditional mashed potatoes, but taste much better than the mashed turnip variation.

📚 When deciding which meal to cook for you child, consider the size of the recipe. There is a moderate variance in portion sizes depending on the amount of carbohydrates in the recipe. Strawberries, blueberries, and apples are very low in carbohydrates, as are green beans and carrots. If your child is especially hungry, offer meal choices with larger portions.

📚 Try to mix the medications into the foods. Do not put seizure medications in before heating meals, as the heat may alter their effectiveness. Cream is an excellent place to hide the meds (using the cream as milk, pudding, or whipped).

📚 Keep in mind that if your child is on Carnitor (a carnitine supplement), he/she may be in a stronger ketosis because of the carnitine itself.

📚 Serving food in store containers can be a special treat. Bryce really liked to have yogurt in the Dannon container. You can transfer the Dannon Light n' Fit Carb and Sugar Control Yogurt into a clean bowl, then wash out the original container and dry. Next, put the Dannon container on the scale and zero it, then measure the yogurt, cream, and oil into the container (see the recipe section for yogurt recipes). Bryce was amused to be eating something he saw at the store and on TV!

✂ Give keto-Popsicles when your child is hungry. Make by pouring keto-Kool-Aid in an ice cube try or Popsicle tray. Place a piece of aluminum foil tightly over the top, cut slits over the middle of each compartment with a knife, then put a Popsicle stick in the slit. Freeze for a few hours. You can make "fancy" Popsicles by using two different colors of keto-Kool-Aid in one Popsicle, or you may even be able to find fancy-shaped ice cube trays. Part of the fun of keto-Popsicles for Bryce was that he didn't have to finish it all (a rare treat for a keto-kid).

✂ Keep in mind when calculating recipes that you don't need to use all of the carbohydrate allotment as carbohydrate. You can go over on the protein and under on the carbohydrate as long as the total protein and carbohydrate is not over the total allotment. Actually, meals with more protein are more ketogenic, and you will notice that they produce a stronger ketosis in your child.

✂ Many snowcone machines at amusement parks only use crushed ice (whereas home snow cone machines require sugar and salt to be added to the ice). Ask when you see a machine at an amusement park; you can pour keto-Kool-Aid over the crushed ice and have a wonderful keto-treat. The best part of all is that it looks exactly like what the other kids are eating!

✂ Have a plan in case your scale breaks! Locate a manufacturer near you where you can get a replacement. Our scale broke after our first year, then broke about three more times after that. You can rely on your freezer food to get you through a day or two until your scale is replaced (because it's already been measured) although you may have to guess on the cream in a pinch.

✂ Consider using sugar-free Jell-O as a free food. One serving is one-quarter of the package and has 1 gram of protein and no carbs! Compare that to a serving of two macaroon cookies (which also use sugar-free Jell-O mix); they have 1 gram of protein and 0.1 grams of carbs. Two macaroon cookies are gone in two bites; even an eighth of the package is a nice serving of sugar-free Jell-O, would have only 0.5 grams of protein, and is a much heartier portion. You can make the sugar-free Jell-O in a rectangular baking dish, or make individual servings in Pyrex glass bowls. You can also get fancy and use holiday shapes and colors throughout the year (ex: red sugar-free Jell-O in a small heart-shaped custard dish for Valentine's Day).

❧ You can make your own keto-candy using candy molds or even ice cube trays. You can also make keto-chocolate suckers this way. I always made them for special occasions (see the recipe section).

❧ The following low-carb foods work well on the ketogenic diet:

- ❧ Dannon Light n' Fit Carb and Sugar Control Yogurt
- ❧ Le Carb Ice Cream (chocolate, vanilla, strawberry)
- ❧ Kix cereal (see the "Breakfast" section of Chapter 4 for other low-carb cereals)
- ❧ Ocean Spray Light Cran-Grape Juice
- ❧ Pepperidge Farms Goldfish Crackers and Baby Goldfish Crackers
- ❧ Teddy Grahams
- ❧ Troyer Farms Corn Puffs, Cheese Puffs, Pretzels, and Potato Chips
- ❧ Dan Dee Corn Twisters
- ❧ Doritos
- ❧ Keto brand Nacho Tortilla Chips
- ❧ Mini-Vanilla Wafers

❧ Use noniodated salt or sea salt. Salt with iodine contains sugar, which may disrupt ketosis.

It cannot be overstated that ketogenic meal preparation absolutely gets easier with time. After a few months, you will be amazed at how much simpler keto-cooking is compared to the first few weeks on the diet! You will also be surprised to find that the extra time it takes to make ketogenic meals just sort of creates itself. You will find the time that you need, and keto-cooking will become a normal way of life for you. By incorporating the above tips into your routine, ketogenic cooking will become less time consuming and less challenging with the passing of each day. The ketogenic diet is the greatest gift that you could ever give your child.

Every ounce of effort is worth it!

CHAPTER 4

KETOGENIC
RECIPES

All of my recipes are based on a meal with 5.5 grams protein, 30 grams fat, and 4.2 grams carbohydrate. As a reference point, they are for a 5-year-old on about 1,100 calories daily. Please use these recipes as a guide only. Do not copy them exactly for your child. Each recipe must be tailored to meet your child's specific protein, fat, and carbohydrate allowance. It is important to remember that the protein, fat, and carbohydrate values vary for different brands of foods.

I highly recommend that you learn to calculate recipes for yourself. It is challenging at first, but in the end will give you and your keto-kid tremendous flexibility in meal planning. Meal calculations get much, much easier over time.

When we started the ketogenic diet, we left the hospital with only about five actual recipes. It was very frustrating to have to calculate the meals while Bryce was hungry and waiting for his food. I would recommend that you preview the recipes below with your child, and mark 10 or 15 of their favorites. Take this book with you to the hospital at the induction of the diet, along with the actual labels of the brands of foods that you plan to use.

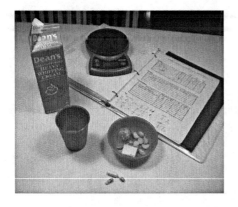

Have your dietician calculate exact recipes specifically for your child before you leave the hospital. This should eliminate the frustration we experienced.

Again, you should not try to exactly copy the ingredient amounts for your child, as the grams of each ingredient will vary with the amount of calories your child is allotted, as well as the breakdown of the protein, fat, and carbohydrate allotment. I have not included the protein, fat, and carbohydrate values from the food labels that I used because this will help prevent you from copying exactly. I strongly believe that providing accurate meals for you child helps achieve successful ketosis and subsequent seizure control. We never used substitution charts for fruits and vegetables because the protein, fat, and carbohydrate values vary so much! I truly believe that our commitment to details and accuracy was partly responsible for our success.

That being said, it was very helpful for me to have a good idea of the ingredient proportions when calculating recipes, which is why I included them here. When you calculate your own recipes, try to keep the proportions of ingredients roughly equivalent. If your child is on a ratio greater than 3:1, you can often just use a little more fat (cream, oil, or butter) to get the appropriate proportions. If your child's ratio is less than 3:1, simply add more carbohydrate or protein (the meat, vegetable, or fruit). You may consider making a few of these recipes before your child starts the ketogenic diet as both practice for you and as a reassurance to your child that they will still be able to enjoy good foods on the ketogenic diet. For practice only, you may use the values below exactly, and the brands don't matter.

BREAKFAST MEALS

Note: In this "Breakfast Meals" section, I have purposefully listed many similar egg recipes, with only the carbohydrates varying in each recipe. (I did not do this in the other sections.) It is importannt to realize that when you change *any* part of the recipe, it *will* affect the remainder of the recipe. To illustrate this point, compare and contrast the egg recipes. If you serve eggs with strawberries rather than with bananas, for example, your child will get about three times as much fruit because strawberries are much lower in carbohydrates than bananas. If you choose "Eggs with Bacon and Orange Juice" rather than "Eggs and Bacon," you will notice that you get less bacon and less eggs in the recipe with the orange juice, but more butter. The reason is that the recipe with orange juice uses less cream (the fat) and adds carbohydrates (the orange juice). You will have remendous flexibility on the ketogenic diet to vary the recipes to match your child's food preferences. Just remember to recalculate your recipes accordingly.

❧ *Apple Eggnog*

Cream: 70 grams
Egg (XL): 32.8 grams
Apple juice: 12.8 grams
Canola oil: 3.8 grams
Liquid sweetener: 20 drops
Vanilla: 5 drops

1. Mix egg whites and yolks together in a bowl, then measure out amount and cook in the microwave about 1 minute or until done.
2. Mix all in a blender.

Hints: Each sip is ketogenically balanced, so this meal would work if your child is sick and not very hungry. (My son, however, preferred muffins or cupcakes on sick days). This meal is also

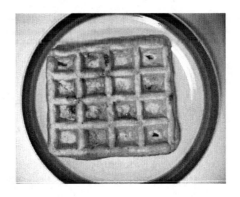

great for travel. Your child can drink it in the car without any major consequences if a drop is spilled or it is not 100% scraped (again, because every sip is ketogenically balanced). It can also be frozen and eaten with a spoon for a special treat.

🌿 Waffles or Pancakes (with Blueberries or Strawberries)

Cream: 10 grams
Blueberries, chopped: 5 grams
Eggbeaters: 38 grams
Planters macadamia nuts, ground: 20 grams
Butter: 7.3 grams
Canola oil: 6 grams
Liquid sweetener: 20 drops

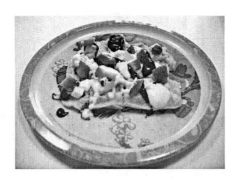

1. Hold the butter and cream; it's not mixed into the pancake.

2. Mix the Eggbeaters, oil, chopped blueberries, ground macadamia nuts, and sweetener in a small mixing bowl with one beater.

3. Pour mixture into a nonstick skillet sprayed with Pam and brown both sides. For waffles, pour mixture into one side of a waffle iron that has been sprayed with Pam.

4. Serve with the butter melted on top and milk to drink, or see the "Ketogenic Cooking" section for the many uses of cream.

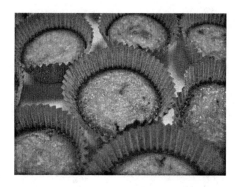

Hints: This is another great recipe to mass produce and freeze. A waffle or pancake can be reheated easily in the toaster oven for 3–6 minutes. I used Walden Farms brand chocolate syrup and pancake syrup and topped the pancakes with a small teaspoon of either. Sometimes I put a teaspoon of the pancake syrup in a small container (the Crystal Light mix containers work well), cut the waffle into four strips, and Bryce then had "waffle strips" to dip. Another variation is to whip the cream and put it on top of the pancake or waffle. For the first several months of his diet (when I did not use processed foods), I added 5 drops of vanilla to the recipe, and no syrup on top. I also have a recipe with strawberries; you could calculate in any fruit that your child likes. (Substitute 10 grams of strawberries for the blueberries, and decrease the Eggbeaters to 36.6 grams for this variation.)

🐾 Macadamia Nut Blueberry Muffins

Planters macadamia nuts, ground: 20 grams
Eggs (XL): 24 grams (x 4 = 96 grams)
Butter: 12.2 grams (x 4 = 48.8 grams)
Cream: 10 grams (x 4 = 40 grams)
Blueberries: 10 grams (x 4 = 40 grams)
Liquid sweetener: 20 drops (x 4 = 80 drops)
Vanilla or maple syrup flavoring (Bickford):
    5 drops (x 4 = 20 drops)
Cream of tartar: ¼ teaspoon for a quadruple recipe

1. Separate 2 eggs from whites and measure the whites. Subtract this from 96 to get the amount of yolks needed. Beat the whites until stiff, then add cream of tartar and beat again.

2. Measure egg yolks, then butter and cream, and mix into egg whites until light and creamy.

3. Add ground macadamia nuts, blueberries, sweetener, and vanilla or maple syrup and mix until creamy.

4. Pour into Reynolds Mini-Muffin Baking Cups that are placed on a flat cookies sheet and presprayed with Pam. One batch makes 6 mini-muffins. Use about 1 teaspoon full each and divide evenly into 24 cups. If the recipe is used in single, place in one Reynolds Large Baking Cup which is placed inside a cupcake pan then sprayed with Pam.

5. Bake for 25 minutes or until golden brown on top and springs back.

Hints: I mass-produced this recipe, but it was not exact when divided by the eye and so not a good idea to mass produce for someone starting the diet. (My son maintained terrific ketosis with the mini-muffins). A better idea for someone new to the diet would be to just mix one large muffin at a time then bake them all at once. I made mini-muffins and used 2 muffins (each

0.8 grams protein, 5 grams fat, and 0.8 grams carbs) along with 3.4 grams butter as a snack. Sometimes I calculated a mini-muffin into a meal as "dessert." I used large muffins for breakfast or for special occasions; they were great for trips and could be eaten easily in the car. They were also great for sick days. Both the mini-muffins and the large muffins can be frozen and later thawed, or even warmed in the toaster oven. I found the silver Reynolds cups much better than the paper cups because the paper cups stick! Also, the mini-muffin cups on a cookie sheet make the muffin flatten out and so look bigger.

❧ Apple Carmel Muffins

Planters macadamia nuts, ground: 20 grams
Eggs (XL): 24 grams
Cream: 10 grams
Apples, finely chopped: 10.1 grams
Butter: 12.2 grams
Liquid sweetener: 20 drops
Carmel flavoring (Bickford): 5 drops
Cream of tartar: small pinch (1/4 tsp if quadrupling the recipe)

Follow exact directions for the blueberry muffins. Each muffin has 0.8 grams protein, 5 grams fat and 0.85 grams carbohydrate.

❧ Hard Boiled Egg and Milk

Boiled egg (XL): 49 grams
Cream: 55 grams
Butter: 9.3 grams OR Oil: 7.3 grams

1. Cut off some white from the hard-boiled egg to get the 49 grams.

2. Serve the butter cut up into squares on toothpicks.

3. See the "Ketogenic Cooking" section for the many uses of cream.

4. If making hot chocolate or pudding, oil can be used instead of the butter because it's hidden well in the drink.

Hints: This was always an Easter favorite. When you dye eggs together, simply buy the type that your keto-kid uses (we always bought XL size). Then, your child can have the thrill of choosing a dyed Easter egg and eating it just like everyone else! Hot chocolate is a great place to mix in medicines or supplements like Carnitor.

❧ Hard Boiled Egg and Bacon

Boiled egg (XL): 56 grams
Cream: 20 grams
Bacon (side pork): 2.4 grams
Butter: 22 grams

1. Prepare egg as above.

2. Microwave bacon on a plate lined and topped with paper towels. Measure the bacon once cooked.

3. Cut the bacon and butter into equal number of tiny pieces and top each piece of butter with bacon to make "butter-bacon sandwiches" as Bryce called them.

❧ Deviled Egg

Hard-boiled egg (XL): 56 grams
Cream: 34 grams
Hellman's mayonnaise: 17 .8 grams
Salt: tiny pinch

1. Measure egg and either cut off some of the white or add a piece of white from another egg to get the 56 grams.

2. Cut egg in half lengthwise and separate white and yolk.

3. Mix yolk and mayonnaise and beat together with a hand frother.

4. Put the mixture back into the white and sprinkle a tiny bit of season salt on top.

Hint: We used metal butter containers for mixing these small quantities; they worked well. They are used to dip butter when eating crab legs or lobster. We purchased a package of four for a dollar from our local dollar store.

✿᠍᠍ *Eggs and Applesauce*

Cream: 20 grams
Egg (XL): 40.8 grams
Mott's Applesauce: 13.7 grams
Butter: 25.1 grams

1. Crack the egg and mix the whites and yolk together with a hand frother.

2. In a small plastic bowl, measure out the egg, then zero the scale and measure the cream into the same bowl and mix together with a hand frother. (Alternately, some of the cream could be saved for milk).

3. Melt the butter in a nonstick skillet, then scramble the egg/cream mixture. The cream just makes the eggs fluffier and mixes well.

4. The applesauce is served separately in a small bowl.

❧ *Eggs and Bacon*

Cream: 30 grams
Egg (XL): 38 grams
Bacon (side pork): 8.4 grams
Butter: 16.7 grams

1. Crack the egg and mix the whites and yolk together with a hand frother.
2. In a small plastic bowl, measure out the egg, then zero the scale and measure 10–20 grams of the cream into the same bowl and mix together with a hand frother.
3. Melt the butter in a nonstick skillet, then scramble the egg/cream mixture.
4. The remainder of the cream is used for milk.
5. Cook side pork in the microwave between layers of paper towels and measure after cooked.

❧ *Eggs and Bacon Smile (No Cream)*

Egg (XL): 50 grams
Bacon (side pork): 7.8 grams
Butter: 28.3 grams

1. Crack the egg and mix the whites and yolk together with a hand frother.
2. In a small plastic bowl, measure out the egg.
3. Melt the butter in a nonstick skillet, then cook the egg as one big flat piece.
4. Cook side pork in the microwave between layers of paper towels and measure after cooked.
5. Use Walden Farm's ketchup to make eyes; arrange the bacon to make the nose and the mouth.

Hint: Compare this recipe to the last one. Without the cream, the butter allotment is much greater, but in this case it's easily absorbed into the eggs. The amount of bacon is very similar.

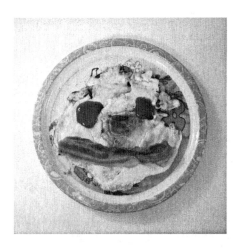

🐾 *Eggs and Bacon with Apple Juice or Applesauce*

Cream: 20 grams
Bacon (side pork): 6 grams
Egg (XL): 24.8 grams
Butter: 23.7 grams
Apple juice: 26.5 grams OR Applesauce: 15.2 grams

1. Crack the egg and mix the whites and yolk together with a hand frother.
2. In a small plastic bowl, measure out the egg, then zero the scale and measure the cream into the same bowl and mix together with a hand frother.
3. Melt the butter in a nonstick skillet, then scramble the egg/cream mixture.
4. Serve with the applesauce in a small bowl OR the apple juice mixed with a few ounces of water in a small cup.

Hint: Mixing the apple juice with water makes it look like more, it still tastes very sweet, especially for our keto-kids who don't get any sugar.

✤ *Eggs and Bacon with Orange Juice*

Cream: 10 grams
Bacon (side pork): 4 grams
Egg (XL): 35.2 grams
Butter: 27.9 grams
Minute Maid Light orange juice: 51.7 grams

1. Crack the egg and mix the whites and yolk together with a hand frother.
2. In a small plastic bowl, measure out the egg, then zero the scale and measure the cream into the same bowl and mix together with a hand frother.
3. Melt the butter in a nonstick skillet, then scramble the egg/cream mixture.
4. Serve with the orange juice mixed with a few ounces of water in a small cup.

Hint: This meal has a lot of variety and is similar to a non-keto breakfast. The orange juice was always a real treat for Bryce.

✤ *Eggs and Orange Juice*

Egg (XL): 38.4 grams
Minute Maid Light orange juice: 51.7 grams
Cream: 20 grams
Butter: 25.3 gram

1. Crack the egg and mix the whites and yolk together with a hand frother.

2. In a small plastic bowl, measure out the egg, then zero the scale and measure the cream into the same bowl and mix together with a hand frother.

3. Melt the butter in a nonstick skillet, then scramble the egg/cream mixture.

4. Serve with the orange juice mixed with a few ounces of water in a small cup.

🍂 Eggs and Oranges

Cream: 30 grams
Egg (XL): 37.6 grams
Orange: 22.4 grams
Butter: 21.3 grams

1. Crack the egg and mix the whites and yolk together with a hand frother.

2. In a small plastic bowl, measure out the egg, then zero the scale and measure 10–20 grams of the cream into the same bowl and mix together with a hand frother.

3. Melt the butter in a nonstick skillet then scramble the egg/cream mixture.

4. The remainder of the cream is used for milk, or see the "Ketogenic Cooking" section for the many uses of cream.

5. Peel the orange and remove any seeds. Meticulously pick off the pulp and choose only the best pieces to measure and cut into tiny slices.

❧ *Eggs and Bananas*

Cream: 30 grams
Bananas: 11.1 grams
Eggs (XL): 38.4 grams
Butter: 21 grams

1. Crack the egg and mix the whites and yolk together with a hand frother.
2. In a small plastic bowl, measure out the egg, then zero the scale and measure 10–20 grams of the cream into the same bowl and mix together with a hand frother.
3. Melt the butter in a nonstick skillet, then scramble the egg/cream mixture.
4. The remainder of the cream is used for milk.
5. Cut the banana into 6–8 tiny slivers. Each one can be served on a toothpick.

Hint: This is a VERY small amount of banana, about a half-inch piece. Nonetheless, my son really missed bananas and so asked for this meal often. He called the banana slivers banana "clones."

❧ *Eggs and Blueberries or Pears*

Cream: 30 grams
Blueberries: 18.1 grams OR Pears 17.2 grams
Egg (XL): 38.4 grams
Butter: 21 grams

1. Crack the egg and mix the whites and yolk together with a hand frother.
2. In a small plastic bowl, measure out the egg, then zero the

scale and measure 10–20 grams of the cream into the same bowl and mix together with a hand frother.

3. Melt the butter in a nonstick skillet, then scramble the egg/cream mixture.

4. See the "Ketogenic Cooking" section for the many uses of cream.

5. Pick through the blueberries to get the smaller ones so that your child gets more. If using pears instead, cut the skin off first, then serve several thin pear slices.

❧ *Eggs and Cheese with Apple Juice or Strawberries*

Cream: 30 grams
Helluva Good sharp cheddar cheese: 28 grams
Egg (XL): 25.6 grams
Butter: 19.6 grams
Apple juice: 21.4 grams
    OR
Strawberries: 32.6 grams

1. Crack the egg and mix the whites and yolk together with a hand frother.

2. In a small plastic bowl, measure out the egg, then zero the scale and measure 10–20 grams of the cream into the same bowl and mix together with a hand frother.

3. Melt the butter in a nonstick skillet, then scramble the egg/cream mixture.

4. See the "Ketogenic Cooking" section for the many uses of cream.

5. Mix the apple juice with water OR cut the strawberries into tiny slices and serve on the side.

Hint: Strawberries are a wonderful keto-food because they are low in carbohydrates and protein; your child will get more strawberries, blueberries, and apples than most other fruits. Sometimes the amount of strawberries is so great that you may even be able to give several whole (small sized) strawberries. This was always very exciting for my son.

This can also be made into a quiche. Mix the egg, cream, butter, and cheese in a small bowl. Spray a small nonstick individual quiche pan and pour in the mixture. Bake at 350 degrees for 30–45 minutes, or until lightly browned on top. This is a great recipe to make ahead and bring on trips or just have on hand in the freezer for a quick breakfast. The apple juice or strawberries would still be served on the side as above.

✌❧ *Eggs and CranGrape Juice*

Egg (XL): 34 grams
Ocean Spray CranGrape Light Juice: 240 grams
Cream: 20 grams
Butter: 25.8 grams

1. Crack the egg and mix the whites and yolk together with a hand frother.
2. In a small plastic bowl, measure out the egg, then zero the scale and measure the cream into the same bowl and mix together with a hand frother.
3. Melt the butter in a nonstick skillet, then scramble the egg/cream mixture.
4. Serve with the CranGrape juice mixed with a few ounces of water in a small cup.

❧ *Eggs and Red Grapes*

Cream: 30 grams
Red grapes: 14.6 grams
Egg (XL): 38.4 grams
Butter: 21 grams

1. Crack the egg and mix the whites and yolk together with a hand frother.
2. In a small plastic bowl, measure out the egg, then zero the scale and measure 10–20 grams of the cream into the same bowl and mix together with a hand frother.
3. Melt the butter in a nonstick skillet, then scramble the egg/cream mixture.
4. See the "Ketogenic Cooking" section for the many uses of cream.
5. Cut the red grapes into slivers and serve on the side.

❧ *Eggs and Strawberries*

Cream: 30 grams
Strawberries: 36.9 grams
Egg (XL): 37.6 grams
Butter: 21 grams

1. Crack the egg and mix the whites and yolk together with a hand frother.
2. In a small plastic bowl, measure out the egg, then zero the scale and measure 10–20 grams of the cream into the same bowl and mix together with a hand frother.
3. Melt the butter in a nonstick skillet, then scramble the egg/cream mixture.
4. See the "Ketogenic Cooking" section for the many uses of cream.

5. Cut the strawberries into slivers or choose small-sized strawberries and serve whole.

Eggs and Watermelon

Cream: 30 grams
Egg (XL): 38.4 grams
Watermelon: 36.2 grams
Butter: 20.9 grams

1. Crack the egg and mix the whites and yolk together with a hand frother.
2. In a small plastic bowl, measure out the egg, then zero the scale and measure 10–20 grams of the cream into the same bowl and mix together with a hand frother.
3. Melt the butter in a nonstick skillet, then scramble the egg/cream mixture.
4. See the "Ketogenic Cooking" section for the many uses of cream.
5. Take the seeds out and cut the watermelon into slivers or choose small sized piece and serve whole.

Eggs and Sausage with Apple Juice

Cream: 20 grams
Bob Evans sausage links: 11.2 grams
Egg (XL): 23.2 grams
Butter: 22.7 grams
Motts Apple Juice: 25.6 grams

1. Crack the egg and mix the whites and yolk together with a hand frother.

2. In a small plastic bowl, measure out the egg, then zero the scale and measure the cream into the same bowl and mix together with a hand frother.

3. Melt the butter in a nonstick skillet, then scramble the egg/cream mixture.

4. Sautee the sausage in a small nonstick skillet with about an eighth of an inch of water and a lid. This will steam the sausage and prevent it from drying out. Pat a link dry then measure when it is cooked. Cut into small pieces to serve.

5. Serve with the apple juice mixed with a few ounces of water in a small cup.

Hint: This can also be made into a quiche. Mix the egg, cream, butter, and cooked and crumbled sausage in a small bowl. Spray a small nonstick individual quiche pan and pour in the mixture. Bake at 350 degrees for 30–45 minutes, or until lightly browned on top. This is a great recipe to make ahead and bring on trips or just have on hand in the freezer for a quick breakfast. The apple juice would still be served on the side as above.

❧ *Eggs and Toast*

Egg (XL): 35.2 grams
Irene's gluten bread: 12.5 grams
Cream: 20 grams
Butter: 25.7 grams

1. Crack the egg and mix the whites and yolk together with a hand frother.

2. In a small plastic bowl, measure out the egg, then zero the scale and measure the cream into the same bowl and mix together with a hand frother.

3. Melt the butter in a nonstick skillet, then scramble the egg/cream mixture.

4. Defrost the bread on a paper towel in the microwave for about 20 seconds. Cut a square out of the middle of the bread, then weigh. Keep trimming off the sides until 12.5 grams is reached. Toast the bread lightly *after* it is weighed.

Note: You may choose to hold back on some of the butter in the eggs and save for the top of the toast.

❧ Cold Cereal and Milk

Kix cereal: 6.1 grams (OR other select brands, see below)
Cream: 87.1 grams
Liquid sweetener: 20 drops

1. Measure out the cream and mix in the sweetener.
2. Use about 20 or 30 grams in a bowl with the cereal.
3. Use the remainder of the cream for milk, served on the side in a cup. There's too much cream to put it all in the bowl with the cereal.

Hints: After spending hours in the grocery store isles reading the labels, Kix is the lowest-carb cereal I found. It was a treat for my son to have cereal at all; this gave him about two hand-fuls. This would be a great breakfast to eat in the car; you could put the cereal in a bag and give the milk all in a cup. You could add a pinch of sugar-free Strawberry Jell-O mix or sugar-free Chocolate Pudding mix, or a small teaspoon of Walden Farms Chocolate Syrup to flavor the milk.

Other relatively low-carb cereals that we used and the proportions are as follows:

Post Carb Well Cinnamon Crunch Cereal:
>6.3 grams cereal
>88.9 grams cream

Post Carb Well Golden Crunch Cereal:
>6.2 grams cereal
>89.2 grams cream

Trix 75% Reduced Sugar Cereal:
>5.7 grams cereal
>89.2 grams cream

Cinnamon Toast Crunch 75% Reduced Sugar Cereal:
>6.8 grams cereal
>88.3 grams cream

Captain Crunch Reduced Sugar Cereal:
>6 grams cereal
>89.5 grams cream

Fruity Pebbles Reduced Sugar Cereal:
>6 grams cereal
>89.5 grams cream

Peanut Butter Toast Crunch Reduced Sugar Cereal:
>6.3 grams cereal
>88 grams cream

❧ Quiche: Egg, Bacon, and Cheese

Cream: 30 grams
Cheese: 10 grams
Bacon: 8 grams
Egg (XL): 19 grams
Butter: 15 grams

1. Crack the egg and mix the whites and yolk together with a hand frother.
2. In a small plastic bowl, measure out the egg, 10 grams of the cream, the cooked and crumbled bacon, the butter, and the cheese and mix together with a hand frother.
3. Spray a nonstick small individual quiche pan with Pam and pour the mixture in.
4. Bake at 350 degrees for 30–45 minutes, or until lightly brown on top.

Hint: This is an excellent meal to mass-prepare ahead of time and have on hand in the freezer for a quick breakfast or for trips. It's better than converting the other egg recipes into quiche because it's an all-in-one meal. (There is no need to worry about having to package up a fruit or juice for traveling.)

❧ Cream of Wheat

Instant Cream of Wheat: 12.2 grams
Cream: 20 grams
Butter: 29.7 grams

1. Mix the dry cream of wheat, butter, and cream in a small bowl and cover with plastic wrap.
2. Microwave for 10–15 seconds, or until hot.
3. You can top with a pinch of cinnamon, or a teaspoon of

Walden Farm's chocolate syrup or a teaspoon of Walden Farm's maple syrup for variety.

🍀 *Oatmeal*

Quaker Quick Oats: 11 grams
Cream: 20 grams
Butter: 28.6 grams
Liquid sweetener: 20 drops

1. Weigh all into a small bowl and microwave for 30 seconds or until butter melts.
2. You can top with a pinch of cinnamon or a small teaspoon of Walden Farms maple syrup or chocolate syrup.

Note: This oatmeal is very runny, but is the closest thing I came up with to mimic hot cereal.

MEALS WITH BACON

All references to bacon are really side pork (which is the meat from which bacon is made, before it's smoked or processed). Your local butcher should be able to supply you with side pork. It takes extra work for the butcher, so you may have to explain why you need it. We would buy in bulk—10 to 20 individually wrapped pound packages, sliced thin, every one to two months from Hanson's Freezer Meats (see page 37 for contact information).

✤ Bacon and Apple Pie

Side pork: 15.3 grams
Apples: 24.3 grams
Butter: 23 grams
Cream: 20 grams
Cinnamon: tiny pinch

1. Microwave the bacon on a plate between layers of paper towels until crisp. Measure the bacon after it is cooked.
2. Dice the apples and put into a plastic bowl with the butter and the cinnamon. Cover with plastic wrap and microwave for 15–20 seconds or until the butter is melted. This is the "apple pie."
3. Top the apple pie with whipped cream, or serve the cream as milk instead. See the "Ketogenic Cooking" section for other uses for cream.

Hint: Care needs to be taken when eating this meal. The apples "swim" in the butter and so it is easily spilled. It's very good, though, and the rest of our family would often have "apple pie" with Bryce (with more apples and less butter).

✤ Bacon and Yogurt Swirl

Cream: 30 grams
Side pork: 13 grams
Dannon Light n' Fit Carb and Sugar Control Yogurt:
    56.5 grams
Canola oil: 13.1 grams

1. Mix yogurt, cream, and oil with a frother.
2. Put 2–3 drops of different food coloring on top of mixture, and swirl (to look like store-bought kids' yogurt).

3. Microwave the bacon on a plate between layers of paper towels until crisp. Measure the bacon after it is cooked.

Hints: The yogurt is processed, so not for all keto-kids and not for beginners on the diet. This was also one of my son's favorites. You can freeze the yogurt for a "frozen yogurt" treat. It's a nice-sized portion and filling. We did add a little noniodized salt to the bacon after it was cooked. For a variation, you could calculate pepperoni instead of the bacon, but do this only if your child is able to tolerate processed foods (pepperoni is processed and side pork is not).

🐖 *Bacon and Chocolate Pudding*

Cream: 50 grams
Side pork, sliced thin and microwaved until crisp:
   21.6 grams
Canola oil: 4.3 grams
Liquid sweetener: 20 drops

1. Whip the cream with a hand frother, then add sweetener, oil and one small teaspoon of Walden Farms chocolate syrup and whip again.
2. Microwave the bacon on a plate between layers of paper towels until crisp. Measure the bacon after it is cooked.

Hints: This is not processed (except for the Walden Farms chocolate syrup) and so is pretty keto-friendly. If new on the diet, you could use a pinch of sugar-free Jell-O mix to make a flavored pudding instead. This is also a very large meal.

❧ *Bacon with Bean and Carrot Blend*

Cream: 10 grams
Side pork: 13.5 grams
Birds Eye bean/carrot blend: 65.5 grams
Butter: 26.9 grams

1. Microwave the bacon on a plate between layers of paper towels until crisp. Measure the bacon after it is cooked.
2. Steam the vegetables, pat dry, and measure roughly equal amounts of the beans and carrots.
3. Melt the butter in the measured vegetables. At times we had to microwave the mixture to get the butter to melt.
4. See the "Ketogenic Cooking" section for the many uses of cream."

Hint: This meal gives a lot of vegetables! This can be helpful when your child is first on the diet and hungry. It can be a challenge to get your child to eat all the vegetables if they've been on the diet for awhile and their stomach is small.

❧ *Bacon with Bean and Carrot Blend and One Apple Cookie*

Apple Cookie (see recipe under snacks): #1
Birds Eye bean/carrot blend 60.5 grams
Side pork: 11.1 grams
Butter: 26.7 grams

1. Prepare the bacon and vegetable as above.
2. Serve with one cookie.

Hint: This is a good example of how you can alter your recipes to include treats/desserts or to exclude the cream if your child is tired of the cream.

❧ Bacon with Carrots and One Muffin

Mini blueberry muffin (see recipe under "Breakfast"): #1
Hanover cut carrots: 48.2 grams
Side pork: 12.3 grams
Butter: 25.3 grams

1. Microwave the bacon on a plate between layers of paper towels until crisp. Measure the bacon after it is cooked.
2. Steam the vegetables, pat dry, and measure.
3. Melt the butter in the measured vegetables. At times we had to microwave the mixture to get the butter to melt.
4. Serve with one mini-muffin for dessert.

Hint: This recipe gives a lot of carrots. We always made Bryce eat the bacon and carrots first, before he got the mini-muffin. This really helped him to eat without complaining. If you'd like, some of the butter could be set aside to top the mini-muffin.

❧ Bacon with Carrots, Milk, and One Muffin

Cream: 10 grams
Mini blueberry muffin (see recipe under "Breakfast"): #1
Carrots: 43.9 grams
Side pork: 12 grams
Butter: 21.3 grams

1. Prepare bacon and carrots as above.
2. Serve with one mini-muffin.
3. See the "Ketogenic Cooking" section for the many uses of cream.

Hint: This recipe compared to the one above is a good example of how we would compromise with Bryce. It was created after he complained that there were too many carrots to eat. You can easily alter most recipes to suit your child's desires at the time. Here, I added cream. which allowed me to decrease the carrot and butter portions.

🍀 Bacon and Corn

Cream: 20 grams
Hanover premium corn: 19.1 grams
Side pork: 14.1 grams
Butter: 22 grams

1. Microwave the bacon on a plate between layers of paper towels until crisp. Measure the bacon after it is cooked.
2. Steam the vegetables, pat dry, and measure.
3. Melt the butter in the measured vegetables. At times we had to microwave the mixture to get the butter to melt.
4. See the "Ketogenic Cooking"" section for the many uses of cream.

Hint: Be careful with brands of frozen corn; they can vary widely in carbohydrate values. We found this corn to be the lowest in carbohydrates, thus allowing a larger portion. It's still only a few teaspoons of corn.

🍀 Bacon and Corn with One Muffin

Cream: 10 grams
Mini blueberry muffin: #1
Hanover premium corn: 19.1 grams
Side pork: 12.3 grams
Butter: 21 grams

1. Prepare bacon and corn as above.
2. Serve with one muffin.
3. See the "Ketogenic Cooking" section for the many uses of cream.

❧ Bacon and Red Grapes

Butter: 14.3 grams
Bacon: 15 grams
Red grapes: 19.5 grams
Cream: 20 grams

1. Microwave the bacon on a plate between layers of paper towels until crisp. Measure the bacon after it is cooked.
2. Wash the grapes and pat dry. Remove the seeds and cut in half or quarters, then weigh.
3. See the "Ketogenic Cooking" section for the many uses of cream."

❧ Bacon and Green Beans

Cream: 40 grams
Green beans: 60.1 grams
Side pork: 12 grams
Butter: 14.9 grams

1. Microwave the bacon on a plate between layers of paper towels until crisp. Measure the bacon after it is cooked.
2. Steam the vegetables, pat dry, and measure.
3. Melt the butter in the measured vegetables. At times we would have to microwave the mixture to get the butter to melt.

4. See the "Ketogenic Cooking" section for the many uses of cream.

Hint: This is another very large recipe, due to the amount of green beans. It will be helpful if your child is hungry but a challenge if your child has been on the diet awhile and wants small amounts.

✽❧ Bacon and Ice Cream

Cream: 50 grams
Side pork: 21.6 grams
Canola oil: 4.3 grams

1. Microwave the bacon on a plate between layers of paper towels until crisp. Measure the bacon after it is cooked.
2. Mix the oil in the cream, whip, add sweetener and flavoring (ex: 5 drops of Bickford's flavoring or a pinch of sugar-free Jell-O pudding mix), then freeze for ice cream.

Hint: This type of ice cream is great for beginners on the diet. It tastes fairly good, but is different in texture and taste compared to regular ice cream. The ice cream in my snack section uses a processed ice cream as the base and is delicious; however, being processed, it is best used only after seizure control has been achieved.

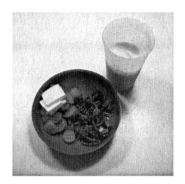 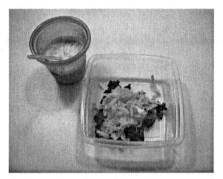

MEALS WITH BEEF

You must be careful to get the same ground beef each time; the protein and fat values vary. After awhile on the diet, we had different recipes for ground round and for 85% lean beef (from two different grocery stores in town). It is easier to use just ONE brand at first, but as your comfort with the diet grows you can use more than one for convenience IF you remember to double-check the protein and fat values each time.

✿❧ *Burger with Cheese*

Ground round beef: 25 grams
Helluva Good cheddar cheese: 10 grams
Cream: 40 grams
Butter: 12.3 grams

1. Brown the beef in a nonstick skillet, pat dry on paper towels, and weigh after cooked.
2. Cube the butter and place on top of the beef.

3. Grate or thinly slice the cheese and layer on top of the butter, then microwave the dish for 10 seconds, or until the butter and cheese are melted.

4. See the "Ketogenic Cooking" section for the many uses of cream.

✿ Burger and Carrots

Cream: 40 grams
Ground round beef: 21.4 grams
Frozen carrots: 42.5 grams
Butter: 17.2 grams

1. Brown the beef in a nonstick skillet, pat dry on paper towels and weigh after cooked.

2. Cube the butter, mix about half into the beef and melt it in the microwave.

3. Steam the vegetables, pat dry, then weigh.

4. Melt the rest of the butter in the vegetables.

5. See the "Ketogenic Cooking" section for the many uses of cream.

✿ Meatballs and Apple Pie

Cream: 20 grams
Apples: 24.3 grams
Ground beef (85% lean): 26 grams
Butter: 24.6 grams
Cinnamon: small pinch

1. Make the beef into meatballs by rolling raw meat into gum-ball-sized balls and boiling for 15–20 minutes or until cooked through. Pat dry on paper towels and weigh after cooked.

2. Peel and dice apples, then weigh. Mix with butter and a small pinch of cinnamon. Cover and microwave for one minute, or until the butter is melted.

3. Whip the cream to top on the apples, or serve as milk. See the "Ketogenic Cooking" section for other uses of cream.

Hint: This is an excellent meal to mass produce ahead of time and put in the freezer for later. Label the container with masking tape to indicate that it is served with 20 grams of cream. Also, consider making meatballs or hamburger for the rest of the family when this meal is served.

🍀 Burger and Blueberries

Cream: 40 grams
Ground beef: 23.4 grams
Blueberries: 21.3 grams
Butter: 16.5 grams

1. Brown the beef in a nonstick skillet, pat dry on paper towels, and weigh after cooked.

2. Cube the butter, mix into the beef, then melt in the microwave.

3. Rinse the blueberries, pat dry, then weigh.

4. Use the cream for milk or whip and use to top the blueberries. See the "Ketogenic Cooking" section for the many uses of cream.

❧ Burger and Green Beans

Cream: 20 grams
Ground round: 21.4 grams
Frozen green beans: 72.9 grams
Butter: 21.4 grams

1. Brown the beef in a nonstick skillet, pat dry on paper towels, and weigh after cooked.
2. Cube the butter, mix about half into the beef, and melt it in the microwave.
3. Steam the vegetables, pat dry, then weigh.
4. Melt the rest of the butter in the vegetables.
5. See the "Ketogenic Cooking" section for the many uses of cream.

Hint: This is a huge amount of green beans, and also a good freezer meal.

❧ Burger and Green Beans with One Muffin

Mini blueberry muffin: #1
Frozen green beans: 56.7 grams
Ground round beef: 18.3 grams
Butter: 25.5 grams
Cream: 20 grams

1. Prepare burger and green beans as above.
2. Serve with one muffin.
3. You may choose to save some of the butter for the muffin.

Hint: This is a good example of compromise. The burger and green beans recipe has a LOT of green beans, so I developed this recipe to lessen the amount. We made Bryce eat all of his beef and green beans before he was allowed to eat the muffin; it helped prevent whining.

🐝 Burger and Green Bean Blend with Two Muffins

Mini blueberry muffin: #2
Birdseye green bean blend: 43.7 grams
Ground round beef: 17.3 grams
Butter: 33.6 grams

1. Prepare the burger and vegetable as above.
2. Serve with TWO muffins.
3. You may choose to save some of the butter for the muffin.

Hint: Bryce suggested this recipe—he optimized his favorite part (the muffin) and minimized his least favorite (the vegetable). Letting your keto-kid give input in this way helps them to take ownership in their diet.

🐝 Burger and Green Bean Blend with Two Muffins and Cream

Mini blueberry muffin: #2
Birsdeye green bean blend: 33.6 grams
Ground round beef: 15.8 grams
Butter: 25.3 grams
Cream: 20 grams

1. Prepare the burger and vegetable as above.
2. Serve with TWO muffins.

3. See the "Ketogenic Cooking" section for the many uses of cream.

Hint: Comparison of the above three recipes also shows the *flexibility* you have with the ketogenic diet. You can vary your recipes slightly to accommodate your needs at the time. For example, recipes with cream are excellent if you child is on medication (meds are easily hidden in cream). Notice also the difference in the butter, ground round and vegetables when adding in a little cream.

❧ Burger, Hot Dog, and Green Beans

Hebrew National hot dog: 25 grams
Wegman's burger (85% lean): 20 grams
Wegman's green beans: 17.8 grams
Butter: 24.9 grams

1. Brown the beef in a nonstick skillet, pat dry on paper towels, and weigh after cooked.
2. Cube the butter, mix about half into the beef, and melt it in the microwave.
3. Steam the vegetables, pat dry, then weigh.
4. Melt the rest of the butter in the vegetables.
5. Wrap one hot dog in a paper towel and microwave for 50 seconds. Pat dry, then cut into small coin-sized pieces and weigh.
6. See the "Ketogenic Cooking" section for the many uses of cream.

Hint: Notice that these brands are different from most of the others I used. I developed this recipe while on vacation, and had to re-calculate everything with the new values. This is a great meal for picnics or vacation and can be mass-produced ahead of time and stored in the freezer. It is especially nice for trips because it doesn't require any cream.

🐾 Burger "Taco"

Doritos: 5 grams
Ground round beef: 24.4 grams
Cream: 30 grams
Butter: 19.1 grams

1. Brown the beef in a nonstick skillet, pat dry on paper towels, and weigh after cooked.

2. Cube the butter, mix into the beef, and then melt it in the microwave.

3. Measure the Doritos in a paper muffin cup and break into ¼ in.-sized pieces.

4. See the "Ketogenic Cooking" section for the many uses of cream.

Hint: Bryce was thrilled with this meal because of the Doritos. Five grams of Doritos works out to be about two chips, but it looks like more if you break them up. I sent this meal to school for Bryce when tacos were served for lunch.

🐾 Bottom Round Roast and Green Beans

Bottom round roast beef: 13.4 grams
Green beans: 56.7 grams
Mini-muffin: #1
Cream: 10 grams
Butter: 25.7 grams

1. Prepare roast by placing in a roasting pan with a little water in the bottom and cook as directed on the package until done. Choose a select cut (from the inside of the roast) and measure.

2. Steam the vegetables, pat dry, then weigh.

3. Melt all but 10 grams of the butter in the vegetables.

4. See "Breakfast" section for mini-muffin recipe. Put the remaining 10 grams of butter on top of the muffin.

5. See the "Ketogenic Cooking" section for the many uses of cream.

Hint: This is a great recipe to use for a family meal; everyone in the family can have the roast beef and the green beans. You can make a few other side dishes for the rest of the family (being mindful not to tempt your keto-kid, of course).

✌ *Top Round Roast with Apple Pie*

Top round roast beef: 15.5 grams
Apples: 22.3 grams
Butter: 24.4 grams
Cream: 30 grams

1. Prepare roast by placing in a roasting pan with a little water in the bottom and cook as directed on the package until done. Choose a select cut (from the inside of the roast) and measure.

2. Peel and dice apples, then weigh. Mix with butter and a small pinch of cinnamon. Cover and microwave for one minute, or until the butter is melted.

3. Whip the cream to top on the apples, or serve as milk. See the "Ketogenic Cooking" section for other uses of cream.

Hint: Note that the values for top and bottom round differ.

MEALS WITH CHICKEN

For all of the recipes below, we boiled boneless, skinless breast of chicken for about 20–30 minutes, or until no longer pink inside. This seemed the best way to prepare the chicken to prevent it from being dry. When measuring the chicken, choose only the choice pieces.

❧ *Chicken with Apple Pie*

Chicken breast: 21.5 grams
Apples: 24.3 grams
Cream: 20 grams
Butter: 29.3 grams
Cinnamon: pinch

1. Measure the chicken and melt about half of the butter over it.

2. Cube the apple (no skin) and put in a microwavable dish. Add the rest of the butter and a pinch of cinnamon. Cover and microwave about 15 seconds, or until butter is melted.

3. Whip the cream (with a few drops of liquid saccharin) and use as whipped cream, or make ahead and freeze and serve as ice cream on top of the apple pie.

❧ *Chicken Nuggets and Carrots (or Corn)*

Bakin Miracle: 4 grams
Hanover frozen sliced carrots:
    31.2 grams (or Birdseye corn: 10.4 gramsc
Chicken: 20 grams
Butter: 36.8 grams

1. Measure the chicken and cut into strips.

2. Dip chicken strips into water then Bakin Miracle and place on a microwave-safe plate.

3. Microwave for about 20–30 seconds.

4. Serve the butter with the vegetable, or hold some butter out to make a "butterball" for dessert (butter rolled into a ball, dipped in water with flavoring and sweetener and frozen).

Hints: This is the lowest carb breading I've found; it's pretty tasty and now the whole family uses it. The amount of chicken is overall small (similar to most keto-recipes) but what kid doesn't love chicken nuggets, so it's worth it!

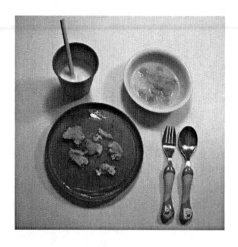

❧ Chicken Nuggets with Carrots and Milk

Bakin Miracle: 4 grams
Cream: 20 grams
Hanover frozen sliced carrots: 22.7 grams
Chicken: 18.7 grams
Butter: 28.4 grams

1. Measure the chicken and cut into strips.
2. Dip chicken strips into water then Bakin Miracle and place on a microwave-safe plate.
3. Microwave for about 20–30 seconds.
4. Serve the butter with the vegetable, or hold some butter out to make a "butterball" for dessert (butter rolled into a ball, dipped in water with flavoring and sweetener and frozen).
5. See the "Ketogenic Cooking" section for the many uses of cream.

❧ Chicken Nuggets with Strawberries

Chicken: 25 grams
Cream: 40 grams
Bakin Miracle: 4 grams
Strawberries: 17 grams
Canola oil: 15.6 grams

1. Measure the chicken and cut into strips.
2. Dip chicken strips into water then Bakin Miracle.
3. Use 8 grams of the oil to fry the chicken strips, then transfer to a plate. Remember to use a spatula to the frying pan when done and scrape every drop of oil back onto the top of the fried chicken strips.
4. Use the remaining 7.6 grams of oil by combining with the cream, adding a few drops of liquid saccharin and a pinch

of sugar-free Jell-O mix or a small teaspoon of Walden Farms chocolate syrup and whipping to make pudding.

❧ Chicken, Cheese, and Bacon

Chicken: 22 grams
Helluva Good sharp cheddar cheese: 6 grams
Side pork: 6 grams
Cream: 20 grams
Butter: 23.8 grams

1. Layer the chicken, butter, side pork, then cheese into a microwave-safe dish, then microwave for about 20 seconds, or until butter and cheese are melted.
2. See the "Ketogenic Cooking" section for the many uses of cream.

Hint: Pyrex bowls work great for this dish. This is an excellent dish to prepare in mass quantities and freeze for future use.

❧ Chicken and Applesauce

Chicken: 22 grams
Applesauce: 17.1 grams
Cream: 20 grams
Butter: 18.2 grams

1. Measure the chicken and melt the butter over it.
2. Serve with milk.

Hint: This is a basic ketogenic recipe and excellent for the first few months of the diet. You can calculate a similar recipe using any fruit or vegetable instead of the applesauce. Later on in the diet, you can recalculate the recipe to add one or two mini-muffins or a cookie for dessert.

✌ Chicken Noodle Soup and Milk

Chicken bouillon: 3.7 grams (1 cube)
Zucchini: 40 grams
Carrots: 15.6 grams
Chicken: 18.1 grams
Canola oil: 19.7 grams
Cream: 30 grams

1. Peel the skin off a zucchini with a vegetable peeler. Then you can use the peeler to slice the zucchini for "noodles" or cut with a knife to make strips. Try not to use the seeds. Place the zucchini in a microwave-safe bowl, cover with plastic wrap, then microwave for 2–3 minutes (depending on the amount of zucchini you cook at once. Lay two clean dish towels on your counter and pour the steamed zucchini onto them; use a third dish towel on top and press to soak up the water. Measure the steamed, dry zucchini into an individual serving-sized bowl.

2. Place a handful of frozen carrots in a microwave-safe bowl, add water, and cover with plastic wrap. Cook in the microwave for 1–2 minutes (or prepare on the stove). Pat the carrots dry before measuring.

3. Mix the zucchini, carrots, chicken, oil, and bouillon cube in the individual serving bowl (like a Pyrex bowl) and add ½ to 1 cup water, then microwave about 45 seconds to heat.

4. See the "Ketogenic Cooking" section for the many uses of cream.

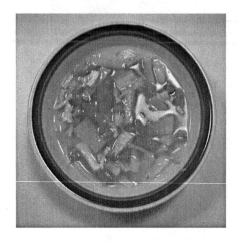

Hints: This recipe contains a lot of liquid; you may have to modify the amount of water used. Your child must finish every last drop of the broth, because it contains a lot of the fat (oil) which is the most important part of a ketogenic meal. It is very tasty and looks exactly like canned soup. It is great to prepare ahead of time and freeze for sick days.

❧ Chicken and Cheese

Chicken: 22 grams
Helluva Good cheddar cheese: 12.8 grams
Cream: 20 grams
Butter: 24.2 grams

1. Layer the chicken, butter and cheese in a microwavable bowl and heat for 20 seconds, or until melted. Mix together.

2. See the "Ketogenic Cooking" section for the many uses of cream.

MEALS WITH HAM AND PORK

Ham is processed and so not tolerated by all keto-kids. It is best to avoid processed foods until seizure control has been achieved, then use sparingly as tolerated by your child.

🎇 *Ham and Apple Pie*

Good Taste ham: 38 grams
Apples: 14.9 grams
Butter: 36.9 grams
Cinnamon: small pinch

1. Cook the ham and then choose the choice cut to measure.
2. Cube the apples, add the butter and cinnamon, and cover with plastic wrap. Microwave for 10 seconds, or until butter is melted.

Hint: Because this meal is all-in-one, it's excellent to mass produce and freeze. For a variation, you can use any vegetable instead of the apples. You could also modify the recipe by adding 10–30 grams of cream (especially if you need a place to hide meds).

🎇 *Pork Chops, Apple Pie, and Macaroon Cookies*

Macaroon cookies: #2 (see recipe on page 115)
Pork chop: 12.8 grams
Apple: 23.6 grams
Butter: 27.9 grams
Cream: 20 grams
Cinnamon: small pinch

1. Spray a baking dish with Pam and bake the pork chop. Once baked, pat the grease off with a paper towel and measure the choice piece.

2. Cube the apples, add the butter and cinnamon and cover with plastic wrap. Microwave for 10 seconds, or until butter is melted.

Hint: For a variation, you can use any vegetable instead of the apples. This recipe is an excellent example of a meal that the whole family can enjoy together!

MEALS WITH HOT DOGS
(AND OTHER PROCESSED MEATS)

Hot dogs are processed and therefore are not to be used during the first month or two on the ketogenic diet. After seizure control has been achieved, you can add in processed foods as tolerated. (You'll know if they are tolerated by whether or not your child seizes after eating processed foods, and whether or not the ketones drop after eating processed foods). We always measured the hot dog after it was cooked, just like all other meats.

✖ *Hot Dog and Apple Pie*
Hebrew National hot dog: 40.8 grams
Apple: 27 grams
Butter: 23.2 grams
Cinnamon: small pinch

1. Wrap the hot dog in a paper towel and microwave for 45–50 seconds.
2. Cube the apples, add the butter and cinnamon, and cover with plastic wrap. Microwave for 10 seconds, or until butter is melted.

Hint: For a variation, you can use any vegetable instead of the apples (hot dog and corn was a favorite of Bryce's). Like all other recipes, you can also add cream if needed or desired. Additionally, for a special treat you could calculate two mini-muffins or a cookie into the recipe.

✽ Hot Dog, Burger and Green Beans

Hebrew National hot dog: 25 grams
Ground round beef: 25.5 grams
Green beans: 20 grams
Butter: 24.2 grams

1. Wrap the hot dog in a paper towel and microwave for 45–50 seconds.
2. Brown the beef in a nonstick skillet, pat dry on paper towels, and weigh after cooked.
3. Steam the vegetables, pat dry and measure.
4. Melt the butter in the measured vegetables. At times we had to microwave the mixture to get the butter to melt.

Hint: This meal was a favorite for cook-outs in the summer. It's a large portion and always left Bryce full. It waa a treat to have two meats at one meal. It worked great to mass-produce and freeze for later use.

Hot Dog, Green Beans, and Mashed Potatoes

Hebrew National hot dog: 40.8 grams
Red-skinned potatoes: 10 grams
Green beans: 18.2 grams
Cream: 20 grams
Butter: 14.8 grams
Salt and pepper: dash

1. For the potatoes, use 10 grams of the cream and 7 grams of the butter. Boil the potatoes, skin and then measure out 10 grams. Whip the potatoes, butter, cream, salt, and pepper with a frother.
2. Wrap the hot dog in a paper towel and microwave for 45–50 seconds.
3. Steam the vegetables, pat dry, and measure.
4. Melt the remainder of the butter in the measured vegetables. At times we had to microwave the mixture to get the butter to melt.

Hint: Bryce liked this meal at holidays; I always made mashed potatoes and green beans for the rest of the family when I made this meal so Bryce felt included.

Kielbasa and Corn

Hillshire Farms kielbasa: 35 grams
Hanover corn: 15.5 grams
Butter: 31.8 grams

1. Pan fry the kielbasa, pat dry, and measure.
2. Steam the vegetables, pat dry, and measure.
3. Melt the butter in the measured vegetables. At times we had to microwave the mixture to get the butter to melt.

Hint: This is another example of a meal that the whole family can eat together. Also, the portion of kielbasa is fairly large.

❧ *Smoked Sausage, Peas, and Carrots*

Hillshire Farms smoked sausage: 30 grams
Shop N Save frozen peas and carrots: 24.6 grams
Cream: 30 grams
Butter: 13.4 grams

1. Pan fry the sausage, pat dry, and measure.
2. Steam the vegetables, pat dry, and measure.
3. Melt the butter in the measured vegetables. At times we had to microwave the mixture to get the butter to melt.
4. See the "Ketogenic Cooking" section for the many uses of cream.

❧ *Bologna and Strawberries*

Oscar Meyer beef bologna: 38 grams
Cream: 56.2 grams
Strawberries: 29.8 grams

1. Weigh the bologna and roll into cylindrical rolls, securing with a fancy toothpick (38 grams is equivalent to roughly two slices).
2. Cut the strawberries into slices or quarters, rinse, pat dry, then measure. The strawberries can also be eaten with a fancy toothpick.
3. Use the cream for milk or for whipped cream on top of the strawberries.

Hint: This was a favorite summer meal for Bryce. It was a nice change from the butter saturated meals and light enough for a hot summer day!

MEALS WITH SEAFOOD

✿❧ *Shrimp with Mandarin Oranges*

Canned mandarin oranges: 26.6 grams
Frozen mini salad shrimp: 46.8 grams
Minced garlic: 2 grams
Butter: 38.2 grams

1. Drain the oranges and pat a few dry. Measure.
2. Thaw the shrimp by running under cold water and pat dry. Measure.
3. Sautee the shrimp in the butter and garlic in a nonstick skillet. Remember to scrape every last drop of butter out of the skillet and back into the serving dish.

✿❧ *Snow Crab Legs with Green Beans and Pudding*

Snow crab legs: 36.4 grams
Green beans: 10.1 grams
Butter: 12.2 grams
Cream: 30 grams
Canola oil: 10 grams

1. Steam the snow crab legs, or better yet have them steamed for you at the grocery store. Crack open and measure.

2. Measure the butter and melt in a small container for dipping (we bought stainless steel seafood butter cups from our dollar store).

3. Steam the vegetables, pat dry, and measure.

4. Whip the cream, then add the oil and a pinch of sugar-free Jell-O mix or a small teaspoon of Walden Farm's chocolate syrup and whip again. Serve for dessert.

Hint: This meal is large and heavy on the protein. It's very nutritious! Notice that I used some oil instead of all butter so that I could hide it in the pudding. For a variation, you could calculate a substitution of any fruit or vegetable for the green beans.

MEALS WITH TURKEY

You must carefully compare turkey labels at your grocery store. Many brands have added sugar or are packed in sugar. We often purchased fresh turkey breast to avoid this. Turkey is very low in protein and fat, so the portions tend to be larger compared with other meats.

✨ *Turkey Breast with Carrots*

Turkey breast: 16.7 grams
Carrots: 40 grams
Butter: 37.4 grams

1. Prepare the turkey with adding only minimal seasonings (like a few pinches of salt, pepper, and Italian seasoning). When

I used a turkey bag, I added flour to the bag to avoid explosion; however, after I coated the bag I dumped the extra flour into the garbage.

2. Select a choice cut of turkey from the inside of the bird to avoid any seasonings or flour in your child's serving. Measure.

3. Steam the vegetables, pat dry, and measure.

4. Use some of the butter on the turkey and the rest for the carrots. Heat in the microwave for about 10 seconds, or until the butter is melted.

Hint: You can calculate a substitution of any vegetable with this meal. This is an excellent meal that the whole family can enjoy—simply add a few side dishes for the rest of the family (preferable ones that your keto-kid doesn't care for).

✷ Turkey and Oranges

Turkey breast: 17.2 grams
Oranges: 25.9 grams
Cream: 40 grams
Butter: 19.5 grams

1. Prepare the turkey with adding only minimal seasonings (like a few pinches of salt, pepper, and Italian seasoning). When I used a turkey bag, I added flour to the bag to avoid explosion; however, after I coated the bag I dumped the extra flour into the garbage.

2. Select a choice cut of turkey from the inside of the bird to avoid any seasonings or flour in your child's serving. Measure.

3. Select choice slices of oranges, and make sure all of the seeds and as much rind as possible is removed. Cut into small pieces, then measure.

4. Measure the butter and melt over the turkey.

5. See the "Ketogenic Cooking" section for the many uses of cream.

Hint: Notice that because I used a fruit instead of a vegetable, I added cream to the recipe to take up some of the fat allotment. Otherwise, the turkey would be swimming in the butter!

❧ *Turkey, Cheese, Bacon, and Milk*

Turkey breast: 27.7 grams
Helluva Good sharp cheddar cheese: 10 grams
Side pork: 6 grams
Cream: 30 grams
Butter: 16 grams

1. Prepare the turkey with adding only minimal seasonings (like a few pinches of salt, pepper, and Italian seasoning). When I used a turkey bag, I added flour to the bag to avoid explosion; however, after I coated the bag I dumped the extra flour into the garbage.
2. Select a choice cut of turkey from the inside of the bird to avoid any seasonings or flour in your child's serving. Measure.
3. Microwave the bacon on a plate between layers of paper towels until crisp. Measure the bacon after it is cooked.
4. Layer the turkey, butter, bacon, and cheese and micro-wave 10 seconds or until the butter and cheese melt.
5. See the "Ketogenic Cooking" section for the many uses of cream.

Hint: This is a very tasty dish and excellent to mass-produce and keep in your freezer. Remember to label the container to state that you must serve with 30 grams of cream.

✌ *Thanksgiving Turkey Meal*

Turkey breast: 21.6 grams
Frozen green beans: 26.3 grams
Idaho potatoes: 10 grams
Cream: 30 grams
Butter: 23.3 grams

1. Prepare the turkey with adding only minimal seasonings (like a few pinches of salt, pepper, and Italian seasoning). When I used a turkey bag, I added flour to the bag to avoid explosion; however, after I coated the bag I dumped the extra flour into the garbage.

2. Select a choice cut of turkey from the inside of the bird to avoid any seasonings or flour in your child's serving. Measure.

3. Skin and cut the potatoes for the entire family. Boil as you normally would. Pat a few pieces dry, and measure 10 grams. Use 10 grams of the cream and 10 grams of the butter and mash together.

4. Steam the vegetables, pat dry, and measure.

5. Melt the remaining butter into the vegetables.

6. Use the remaining cream. See the "Ketogenic Cooking" section for the many uses of cream.

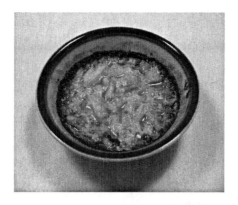

PASTA AND PIZZA MEALS

🎀 *Macaroni and Cheese*

Cooked zucchini: 61.6 grams
Butter: 21.3 grams
Helluva Good sharp cheddar cheese: 22.5 grams
Cream (always Deans heavy whipping cream): 18 grams
Salt (noniodinated) : small pinch

1. Peel a whole zucchini and cut into strips, then further chop into small rectangular pieces (about the size of a macaroni noodle). Microwave the entire cut zucchini on high for 1–2 minutes, until soft. Pour out the excess water, then blot the cooked zucchini on the counter on a dish towel. Weigh the zucchini out in a small glass Pyrex dish that has been sprayed with Pam.

2. In a small plastic bowl, weigh out the butter, cheese, cream and salt then cover with plastic wrap and microwave for 30–60 seconds, or until butter melts.

3. Pour the mixture over the zucchini and mix. Bake in oven at 400 degrees for 20–30 minutes (until the top browns). It's runny, but it will thicken as it cools.

Hints: After getting skilled with the scale, I found it was easier to weigh all the wet ingredients (in step 2) in the same bowl in order to eliminate the ingredients sticking to the side of each separate bowl. I usually mass-produced these in batches of 10 or 15. They freeze well right in the Pyrex bowls (once cooled) then can be thawed in the fridge and microwaved for about a minute to heat. They still may need to set for 5 minutes or so to thicken if re-heated. This tastes wonderful; I ate it myself!

✿ *Spaghetti with Meatballs*

Spaghetti squash, cooked: 54.6 grams
Hunts tomato sauce: 15 grams
Ground round meatballs: 20 grams
Chianti grated parmesan cheese: 3 grams
Butter: 33.1 grams

1. Cut a spaghetti squash lengthwise, scrape out the seeds with a spoon, and place on a cookie sheet face down. Fill the cookie sheet with ¼ inch of water and bake at 350 degrees for about 30 minutes, or until a fork can pass through the rind.

2. Using a fork, scrape lengthwise down the squash to create spaghetti-like pieces. Measure and put in a microwavable bowl.

3. In the meantime, bring water to a boil in a small saucepan. Roll ground round into gumball sized pieces, then drop into the boiling water and cook for about 5 minutes, or until the middle of the meatball is brown. Remove from the water, pat dry, and measure the meatballs.

4. Place the butter and tomato sauce on top of the spaghetti squash and microwave for 10 seconds, or until the butter melts.

5. Top with meatballs then the parmesan cheese.

Hint: This recipe looks just like spaghetti! It's very simple once you get the hang of it, and quite tasty!

(Adapted from "A Family's Guide to the Ketogenic Diet" handbook from Children's Hospital, Pittsburgh, PA.)

❧ *Squash with Cheese Sauce*

Spaghetti squash, cooked: 43.7 grams
Helluva Good cheddar cheese: 14 grams
Chicken breast, boiled: 5.6 grams
Cream: 30 grams
Butter: 23.5 grams

1. Cut a spaghetti squash lengthwise, scrape out the seeds with a spoon, and place on a cookie sheet face down. Fill the cookie sheet with ¼ inch of water and bake at 350 degrees for about 30 minutes, or until a fork can pass through the rind.

2. Using a fork, scrape lengthwise down the squash to create spaghetti-like pieces. Measure and put in a microwavable bowl.

3. Layer the butter, chicken breast and cheese on top and microwave about 20 seconds, or until melted.

4. Serve with cream as milk or pudding.

❧ *Eggplant Parmesean*

Eggplant (cooked): 20 grams
Zucchini (cooked): 53 grams
Hunts tomato sauce: 25 grams
Chicken: 10.8 grams
Pizza cheese: 10 grams
Butter: 34.4 grams

1. Measure a slice of eggplant, and pan fry in a skillet with 15

grams of butter. After browned on each side, transfer to a plate. Take care to scrape every last drop of butter from the skillet back onto the eggplant.

2. Peel the skin off a whole zucchini with a vegetable peeler, then continue to cut into the zucchini with the peeler, making "noodles." Try not to include the seeds. Microwave the zucchini noodles on high for 1–2 minutes, until soft. Pour out the excess water, then blot the cooked zucchini on the counter on a dish towel. Measure the cooked zucchini noodles and place on the plate next to the eggplant.

3. Boil the chicken, pat dry then measure out a choice piece. Place on top of the eggplant.

4. Measure the sauce in a small bowl and add the remainder of the butter; heat in the microwave for 5–10 seconds. Pour the sauce/butter mixture over the "noodles" and eggplant.

6. Sprinkle the cheese over all. Melt it in the microwave for 10 seconds.

Hint: This is not a recipe for beginners! It is one of the most complicated and time-consuming recipes and can be used as a special treat.

❦ Pizza with Pepperoni

Hunts tomato sauce: 10 grams
Planters macadamia nuts, ground: 15 grams
Eggbeaters: 19.3 grams
Hormel beef pepperoni, sliced into eights: 2 grams (1 slice)
Helluva Good sharp cheddar cheese, grated: 12 grams
Canola oil (for crust): 7.5 grams
Canola oil (for sauce): 4.1 grams
Italian seasoning: small pinch

CRUST: Mix Eggbeaters, macadamia nuts, and oil in a small mixing bowl with one mixer. Pour into nonstick skillet sprayed with Pam and brown each side. Transfer onto a paper plate (I used the Zoo pals, to make it fun).

TOPPING: Mix oil, tomato sauce, and small pinch of Italian seasoning in a small container (I used the plastic cups from Crystal Light mix). Spread on pizza, trying to keep the oil from running off the sides. Top with grated cheese and pepperoni.

Hint: These can be mass-produced ahead of time. I placed a piece of wax paper on top of the finished pizza after it cooled, then placed 5–6 pizzas on top of one another in a large freezer bag. Then, at mealtime, I just took from the freezer, removed the wax paper, and microwaved for 30–60 seconds, or until the cheese melted. This pizza looks very similar in size to a personal pan pizza, but is thinner. It is much firmer than the eggplant pizza. It can actually be cut into quarters and picked up to eat (although it's still a little floppier than non-magic pizza). Of course, the toppings can be varied as long as they are calculated into the meal.

SANDWICH MEALS

These recipes are NOT for beginners on the diet. The bread definitely affected my son's ketosis; he was usually in a 3+ rather than a 4+ after eating this bread, but still in a high ketosis so we just limited the bread usage to once a day or once every other day depending on his level of ketosis. All of the recipes use Irene's Gluten Bread, which is made in Cleveland (Irene's Health Bakery, Inc., 11462 Nicholson Road, Garretsville, OH 44231). I buy the bread from Muscarella's Vitamin Center in Hermitage, PA (724-981-1137); the owners Dave and Diane would be happy to ship bread to anyone on the ketogenic diet.

❧ Grilled Cheese

Irene's white gluten bread: 25 grams
Helluva Good sharp cheddar cheese, grated: 9.6 grams
Butter: 34.2 grams

1. Defrost two slices of bread in the microwave, then cut off the crust and weigh, trimming the sides until 25 grams is achieved.
2. Melt the butter in a nonstick skillet.
3. Add the bread, flipping it often to soak up as much butter as possible.
4. After one side is browned, add the cheese and stack the pieces into a sandwich.
5. When browned, transfer to a plate and scrape the remaining butter with a spatula onto the top of the sandwich. It will absorb as it cools.

Hint: This was one of my son's favorites! It works great to take to a restaurant, because grilled cheese is usually on the kids menu.

✤ *Peanut Butter Sandwich*
(WITH BLUEBERRIES, STRAWBERRIES, OR APPLES)

Irene's gluten bread: 25 grams
Peter Pan No Sugar Added peanut butter: 5 grams
Blueberries, sliced: 5 grams (or 10 grams strawberries or
    4.7 grams apples)
Butter: 34.6 grams
Liquid sweetener: 20 drops

1.   Mix butter, sweetener, and peanut butter in a small bowl.

2.   Defrost two slices of bread in the microwave, then cut off the crust and weigh, trimming the sides until 25 grams is achieved.

3.   Initially pile all the peanut butter mixture onto one piece of bread. Use the other piece to scrape the sides of the mixing bowl.

4.   Now divide the peanut butter mixture evenly between the two pieces of bread.

5.   Arrange the sliced fruit on top of the peanut butter on one of the halves, then sandwich together. The fruit acts as the "jelly."

Hints: This is an excellent food for trips. We always took it to the zoo, and packed regular peanut butter sandwiches for the rest of the family. It's nice because it doesn't require any scraping and is an all-in-one recipe. In the summer months, it must be kept in a cooler to avoid the butter melting. As with the grilled cheese sandwich, the bread may affect ketosis so monitor your child closely.

❧ Bologna and Cheese Sandwich

Oscar Meyer beef bologna: 28 grams
Helluva Good cheddar cheese: 4.4 grams
Butter: 32.7 grams
Irene's Gluten Bread: 25 grams

1. Defrost two slices of bread in the microwave, then cut off the crust and weigh, trimming the sides until 25 grams is achieved.
2. Melt the butter in a nonstick skillet.
3. Add the bread, flipping it often to soak up as much butter as possible.
4. After one side is browned, add the cheese and bologna and stack the pieces into a sandwich.
5. When browned, transfer to a plate and scrape the remaining butter with a spatula onto the top of the sandwich. It will absorb as it cools.

Hint: You can also make a grilled turkey and cheese or ham and cheese sandwich this way.

❧ Open-Faced Tuna Sandwich

Canned tuna: 19.3 grams
Irene's gluten bread: 10 grams
Hellman's mayonnaise: 25.7 grams
Cream: 30 grams

1. Drain the tuna and pat several pieces dry. Measure.
2. Mix the tuna and the mayonnaise and set aside.
3. Cut the crust off of a thin slice of bread and measure until you achieve 10 grams. Toast the bread lightly.

4. Spread the tuna/mayo mixture on top of the bread.

5. See the "Ketogenic Cooking" section for the many uses of cream.

SNACKS

All snacks are based on an approximate 1,100 calorie diet with 1.4 grams protein, 12 grams fat and 2.3 grams carbohydrate.

❧ *Ice Cream*
(CHOCOLATE, VANILLA, OR STRAWBERRY)

LeCarb Brand ice cream: 21 grams
Cream: 15 grams
Canola oil: 4.7 grams

1. Measure the ice cream, then add cream and oil and mix with a hand frother,

2. Can be served as is for "soft serve" or refrozen for hard ice cream.

3. Can top with a small teaspoon of Walden Farm's chocolate syrup.

Hints: The ice cream is processed, so not for beginners on the diet. I bought the ice cream from Muscarella's Vitamin Center, phone number given earlier.

❧ *Milk and Cheese*

Cream: 28.5 grams
Helluva Good cheddar cheese: 7.8 grams

1. Cut the cheese into thin sticks, slices or other fun shapes.
2. See the "Ketogenic Cooking" section for the many uses of cream.

❧ *Milk and Blueberries*

Cream: 36 grams
Blueberries: 12 grams

1. Rinse the blueberries, pat dry, then measure.
2. See the "Ketogenic Cooking" section for the many uses of cream.

Hint: This is an excellent basic recipe. You can substitute any fruit for the blueberries and can vary the use of the cream to come up with hundreds of creations! We used different fruit as it was in season; Bryce loved the variety.

❧ *Milk and Cheese Puffs*

Cream: 30 grams
Dandee Corn Twisters: 5.5 grams

1. Measure the Corn Twisters.
2. See the "Ketogenic Cooking" section for the many uses of cream.

Hint: See the "Ketogenic Cooking" section for other low-carb snacks such as Teddy Grahams, potato chips, pretzels, and popcorn puffs. The amount of junk food in this recipe is small—but my son always thought it was a special treat!

🍀 *Half Devilled Egg*

Hillsdale Farms XL egg, boiled: 26 grams
Hellmann's mayonnaise: 12.6 grams
Seasoned salt: small pinch

1. Cut the hard-boiled egg in half lengthwise. Measure by adding or subtracting yolk to get the correct amount.
2. Remove the yolk and mix with the mayonnaise in a small bowl.
3. Spoon the yolk/mayo mixture back into the egg white, being careful to scrape the bowl to get every last drop. Small infant spoons work good for this.
4. Sprinkle as small pinch of seasoned salt on top.

🍀 *Boiled Egg and Pudding*

Hillsdale Farms XL egg, Boiled: 20 grams
Cream: 20 grams
Canola oil: 3.5 grams

1. Cut the hard boiled egg in half lengthwise. Measure by cutting off some of the white to get the correct amount.
2. Use the cream and oil to make pudding (See the "Ketogenic Cooking" section for the many uses of cream). You could also hide this small amount of oil in the cream to make milk; larger amounts of oil do not mix well in the cream.

🍃 *Peanut Butter and Apples*

Peter Pan No-Sugar Added peanut butter: 32 grams
Apples: 8.8 grams
Butter, softened: 10.9 grams

1. Measure the peanut butter into a small mixing bowl and add the butter. Mix well. The butter will easily be "hidden" in the peanut butter while still preserving a great taste!
2. Skin and thinly slice the apples.
3. Let your child dip the apples into the peanut butter, then remember to scrape the peanut butter bowl to get every last drop.

Hint: You can calculate a substitution of celery or carrots instead of the apples. You can also use macadamia-nut butter as a variation (we found it at our local health food store).

🍃 *Bacon with Butter Dip*

Side pork: 6.9 grams
Butter, softened: 7.4 grams
Cream: 10 grams

1. Microwave the bacon on a plate between layers of paper towels until crisp. Measure the bacon after it is cooked.
2. Let your child dip the bacon in the butter.
3. See the "Ketogenic Cooking" section for the many uses of cream.

✖ Apple Chips, Bacon, and Butter

Seneca apple chips: 3.1 grams
Side pork: 4.5 grams
Butter: 11.3 grams

1. Measure the apple chips.
2. Microwave the bacon on a plate between layers of paper towels until crisp. Measure the bacon after it is cooked.
3. Measure the butter and cut into evenly sized small chunks.
4. Serve the butter with a toothpick, as "butter bacon sandwiches" or layer a piece of apple chip, then butter, then bacon.

Hint: We found the apple chips at our local health food store.

✖ Magic Nuts

Macadamia Nuts: 17 grams

Hint: This is a great recipe to take to the movies or on the go. If your child is on medication, you can calculate the recipe to include cream (for us, this equated into 14 grams of macadamia nuts with 12 grams of cream).

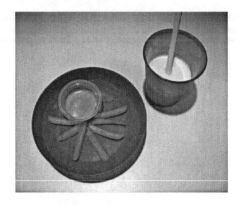

❧ Carrots and Macadamia Nut Butter

Cream: 10 grams
Macadamia nut butter: 8 grams
Carrots, raw: 11.3 grams
Butter, softened: 3.4 grams

1. Mix the jar of macadamia nut butter well before measuring (the nuts and the oil separate during storage). I found this item at Muscarella's (see contact info. under sandwich recipes).

2. Measure the butter, then mix in with the macadamia nut butter.

3. Thinly slice the carrots to use for dipping in the macadamia nut butter mixture. I liked to use the prewashed baby carrots for this recipe.

4. See the "Ketogenic Cooking" section for the many uses of cream.

❧ Apple-Cinnamon Soy Crisps, Bacon, and Butter

Apple-cinnamon soy crisps: 3 grams
Side pork: 4.5 grams
Butter: 12.1 grams

1. Break the soy crisps into quarters and measure.
2. Measure the butter and cut into small cubes (one for each soy crisp).
3. Microwave the bacon on a plate between layers of paper towels until crisp. Measure the bacon after it is cooked.
4. Layer the soy crisps, butter and then bacon on top to make delicious little "sandwich" snacks.

Hint: We found the soy crisps at our local health food store. For a variation, you can substitute Keto Nacho Tortilla Chips (found at our grocery store as well as the health food store).

❧ *Mini-Muffins and Butter*

Mini-muffins: #2 (see recipe in "Breakfast" section)
Butter: 3.2 grams

Hint: I always kept a supply of mini-muffins in the freezer to use for this simple snack or to calculate into a meal for dessert. If you need a place to hide medications, you can calculate a recipe using one mini-muffin, macadamia nuts, butter and cream.

❧ *Apple Carmel Cookies with Milk*

Apple: 4.3 grams
Butter: 9.4 grams
Hillshire Farms XL egg: 10 grams
Nasoya tofu: 11.7 grams
Bickford carmel flavoring: 5 drops
Cream: 10 grams

1. Peel, dice and measure the apples.
2. Mix the egg yolk and white together and measure.

3. Mix all the ingredients together, divide into two, and bake in a muffin pan sprayed with Pam at 350 degrees for 20 minutes or until browned.

4. Let the cookies sit in the muffin pan to cool to allow the butter to soak back in.

5. See the "Ketogenic Cooking" section for the many uses of cream.

Hint: See the dessert section for several other cookie recipes.

❧ *Party Meal*

Strawberries: 20 grams
Watermelon: 20 grams
Carrots: 28.3 grams
Macadamia nut butter: 14 grams
Butter, softened: 24.6 grams

1. Rinse the strawberries, pat dry, slice, then measure.
2. Pick the seeds out of the watermelon, cut, and measure.
3. Rinse the carrots, pat dry, thinly slice, then measure.
4. In a small container, mix the macadamia nut butter and butter until creamy.
5. Have your child use the carrots to dip into the macadamia-nut butter, and serve the fruit with colorful tooth picks.

Hint: I created this meal to simulate the foods served at a friend's birthday party. It would also be great on a hot summer day. You could substitute Peter Pan No Sugar peanut Butter for the macadamia nut butter (the latter which is available at health food stores).

DESSERTS

These desserts would not normally be served as extras, but rather as the meal itself on special occasions.

❧ *Cheesecake with Strawberries (or Blueberries)*

Philadelphia cream cheese: 32 grams
Breakstone sour cream: 12 grams
Eggbeaters: 20 grams
Cream for cheesecake: 20 grams
Cream for topping: 20 grams
Butter: 5.5 grams
Strawberries: 14 grams (or 7 grams blueberries)
Liquid sweetener: 40 drops

1. Spray a small Pyrex bowl with Pam.
2. Measure all ingredients in a microwave-safe bowl, then microwave for about 1 minute or until all ingredients are melted.
3. You can chop up the fruit and mix it in also, or hold it for the topping.
4. Remove from microwave and mix together with a spatula, then pour into the Pyrex bowl.
5. Bake uncovered at 350 degrees for about 30 minutes, or until browned.
6. After it has cooled, whip the cream and a few drops of sweetener and place on top (and fruit if not put inside).
7. You can also drip a small teaspoon of Walden Farms chocolate syrup on top to make it extra fancy. If not using the chocolate syrup, you could add 5 drops of vanilla to the recipe instead.

Hints: This is a great recipe to mass-produce. I find it very good for parties, holidays and sick days. You can make a "swirl" by adding a few drops of food coloring to the cheesecake after you transfer it to the Pyrex bowl; then swirl the food coloring around. You can also color the entire cheesecake or just the whipped cream to match colors used for each holiday. The cheesecake freezes well; just leave out in the fridge the night before needed or defrost in the microwave. I always freeze the cheesecakes without the toppings to keep the whipped cream stiff. A variation would be to add about 10 grams of ground macadamia nuts for a "crust" on the bottom of the bowl (of course, the rest of the ingredients would be recalculated to accommodate the crust).

❧ Chocolate Cupcake with Whipped Cream

Eggbeaters: 10 grams
Cream for cupcake: 5grams
Cream for topping: 10 grams
Butter: 7 grams
Planters macadamia nuts, ground: 24 grams
Sugar-free chocolate Jell-O pudding mix: 3.5 grams
Bickford chocolate flavor: 5 drops
Liquid sweetener: 40 drops
Baking soda: small pinch

1. Whip Eggbeaters and butter.
2. Add nuts, then cream, flavoring, sweetener, and baking soda, and then whip again.
3. Add pudding mix and mix slowly at first, so as not to make the powder blow away.
4. Place a muffin cup into a muffin pan or Pyrex small glass

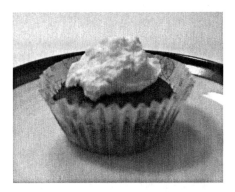

dish, then spray with Pam. (I found Reynolds Large Baking Cups to be the best—silver color—because they don't stick.)

5. Pour mixture into muffin cup and bake at 375 degrees for about 40 minutes.

6. After they have cooled, top with whipped cream.

Hints: This is an excellent birthday or holiday treat! I sometimes topped with a crushed macadamia nut or even dripped a teaspoonful of Walden Farms chocolate syrup on the top. I often put holiday toothpicks in the cupcake. These look very similar to real chocolate cupcakes; I've made Duncan Hines cupcakes for my son's class for his birthday, and it was hard to tell them apart. As a variation, you can use vanilla or strawberry sugar-free Jell-O mix instead to make vanilla or strawberry cupcakes.

✿❦ *Macaroon Cookies*

2 egg whites
1/2 tsp. cream of tartar
1/2 package sugar-free Jell-O

1. Beat egg white until stiff. Add cream of tartar and dry Jell-O.

2. Drop on aluminum foil sprayed lightly with nonstick cooking spray.

3. Bake at 325 degrees for 6–8 minutes, until brown. Cool before eating. Makes 20 cookies. One serving of two cookies contains 1.0 grams protein, 0 grams fat, 0.1 grams carbohydrate.

(From *The Ketogenic Diet: A Treatment for Children with Epilepsy, Fourth Edition,* by John M. Freeman, Eric H. Kossoff, Jennifer B. Freeman, and Millicent T. Kelly. Reprinted by permission of the publisher, Demos Medical Publishing, New York.)

❧ *Muffins–Blueberry or Apple–Caramel*
See "Breakfast" section

❧ *Pumpkin Pie*
Flavorite canned pumpkin: 80 grams
Cream: 60 grams
Butter: 12.3 grams
Liquid sweetener: 30 drops
Vanilla: 5 drops
Cinnamon: small pinch

1. Whip all of the cream. Use 40 grams of the whipped cream in the pumpkin pie and 20 grams for the topping.

2. Combine the 40 grams of whipped cream along with the other ingredients in a mixing bowl and whip together.

3. Pour the mixture in a small Pyrex dish sprayed with Pam.

4. Fill a shallow baking pan with about ¼ inch of water, and place the Pyrex dish on top of it. Bake at 350 degrees for about 30 minutes, or until edges start to brown.

5. After it has cooled, top with the remaining whipped cream.

Note: This is a very large portion. You may even consider using only half the serving, and using the remaining calories for turkey and green beans, or another favorite.

(Adapted from "A Family's Guide to the Ketogenic Diet" handbook from Children's Hospital, Pittsburgh, PA.)

❧ *Chocolate Chip Cookies*

NOTE: THIS IS A SNACK PORTION (1.4 GRAMS PROTEIN, 12 GRAMS FAT AND 2.3 GRAMS CARBOHYDRATE).

Nestle semi-sweet mini morsels: 1.9 grams
Planters macadamia nuts, ground: 9.3 grams
Eggbeaters: 4.1 grams
Butter: 5.7 gram
Liquid saccharin: 40 drops
Salt: small pinch
Baking soda: small pinch
Baking powder: small pinch
Vanilla: 5 drops

1. Measure all ingredients except chocolate chips into a mixing bowl and mix using one electric beater.
2. Use your fingers to scrape the batter off the beater, then add chocolate chips and mix with a spatula.
3. Divide the batter into two equal parts, and put directly in two spots on a muffin pan that have been pre-sprayed with Pam. Remember to scrape the mixing bowl with a spatula to get every last drop.
4. Bake at 350 degrees for 10–15 minutes, or until the edges are browned. Let sit for 5–10 minutes before removing from the muffin tray so that the butter and oil have time to soak back into the cookies.

Hints: I never multiplied this recipe to mass-produce, because most of the carbohydrate allotment is in the chocolate chips and

I didn't want to misjudge and have some of the cookies ending up with too much carbohydrates (thus making then non-ketogenic). Instead, I would prepare the batter for a pair of cookies at a time, then use the same mixing bowl and prepare another pair and bake all at once. When doing this, you must package the correct pairs together so that each pair of cookies remains ketogenically balanced.

❧ Peanut Butter Cookies

A SNACK PORTION.

Peter Pan No-Sugar peanut butter: 5 grams
Eggbeaters: 7.1 grams
Butter: 3.1 grams
Canola oil: 3 grams
Planters macadamia nuts, ground: 5 grams
Liquid sweetener: 20 drops
Baking soda: small pinch
Baking powder: small pinch
Salt: small pinch

1. Measure all ingredients into a mixing bowl and mix using one electric beater.

2. Use your fingers to scrape the batter off the beater.

3. Divide the batter into two equal parts, and put directly in two spots on a muffin pan that have been pre-sprayed with Pam. Remember to scrape the mixing bowl with a spatula to get every last drop.

4. Bake at 350 degrees for 10–15 minutes, or until the edges are browned. Let sit for 5–10 minutes before removing from the muffin tray so that the butter and oil have time to soak back into the cookies.

Hint: You can easily mass-produce this recipe since all ingredients are mixed together and therefore each bite is ketogenically balanced. I multiplied the amounts by six to make a total of 12 cookies at one time.

✌ *Peanut Butter Cups*

A SNACK PORTION.

Peter Pan No-Sugar peanut butter: 8.8 grams
Butter, softened: 8.9 grams
Liquid saccharin: 6 drops
Walden Farms chocolate syrup: one drop

1. Spray a small metal cup or ice cube tray with Pam.
2. Stir the butter, sweetener, and chocolate syrup, and place in a small metal cup. Use your finger to make a little "ditch" in the middle.
3. Place the peanut butter in the "ditch" and freeze.
4. When it has frozen, pop the peanut butter cup out of the container.

Hint: This tastes just like a Reese's Peanut Butter Cup!

✌ *Chocolate Truffles*

A SNACK PORTION

Cream: 106 grams
Bakers unsweetened chocolate: 28 grams
Butter: 25.3 grams
Liquid sweetener: 12 grams
Bickford chocolate flavoring: 4 grams
Ground macadamia nuts: optional

1. In a nonstick saucepan, bring cream to a boil.

2. Stir in chocolate until melted then remove from heat.

3. Add liquid sweetener, butter, and chocolate flavoring, and mix until smooth.

4. Transfer to a cereal-sized bowl and refrigerate for 2 hours, until cool.

5. Scoop a small teaspoon full and roll into a ball; you can then roll in ground macadamia nuts if desired.

Hints: These treats are in a 4:1 ratio. For a 6-gram truffle (without the nuts), there is 0.2 grams protein, 2.4 grams fat, and 0.4 grams carbohydrate, for a total of 26.2 calories. My son absolutely loved these! I sometimes used them as a free food, but ask your dietician first before doing so.

Chocolate for Suckers

Cream: 106 grams
Baker's semi-sweet chocolate: 7 grams
Baker's unsweetened chocolate: 14 grams
Butter: 25.3 grams
Liquid sweetener: 11 grams
Bickford chocolate flavoring: 3 grams

1. In a nonstick saucepan, bring cream to a boil.

2. Stir in chocolate until melted, then remove from heat

3. Add liquid sweetener, butter, and chocolate flavoring, and mix until smooth.

4. Pour into candy molds that have been sprayed with Pam, then freeze.

Hint: These taste very similar to chocolate candy. You can buy holiday sucker or candy molds and matching foil papers from your local craft or baking good store. They must be eaten quickly after removing from the freezer or they will melt. Bryce once told his kindergarten teacher that the Easter Bunny peeked while I was making his magic-candy to learn how! Per one 4 gram serving, there is 0.1 grams protein, 1.6 grams fat, and 0.3 grams carbohydrate. This yields 16 total calories at a 4:1 ratio. I often gave Bryce one or two treats on holidays as his free food for the day, but check with your dietician before doing so.

CHAPTER 5

DAY-TO-DAY REALITIES OF THE KETOGENIC DIET

*E*very family comes to the ketogenic diet from a different group of circumstances. What we all have in common is the tremendous love we have for our keto-kids, and our heartfelt desire to do whatever it takes to make them well. Early on in the diet, we share the struggles inherent in the diet, such as watching our children go hungry and telling them "no" when they ask for the treats that they see other kids enjoying. After some time passes, we share in the joy that reduced seizures or even seizure-free days bring and the hope for a more "normal" future.

My family situation was this: My son Bryce began to seize shortly after his fourth birthday, and within months his epilepsy had progressed to a state uncontrollable by medications. He was having up to 25 seizures daily, including tonic seizures, myoclonic jerks, and atypical absence seizures. I was already more than 4 months pregnant with my second child when Bryce first began to seize. We were blessed to initiate the ketogenic diet early in the course of his epilepsy (which I truly feel is partly responsible for our success). Three weeks after we began the diet, our daughter Grace was born.

One of the ways I coped with Bryce's illness was to write a journal. It was my emotional release. When I re-read my journal now, it brings back my memories vividly, almost too vividly at times. It is amazing to see the progress that we all made, both regarding the physical changes and the emotional changes that the ketogenic diet brings. The diet was much easier for all of us the second year. It will be for you, too.

There is so little information available regarding the day-to-day realities of the ketogenic diet, which is partly what inspired this book. My husband and I read everything we could get our hands on, and still did not have a true grasp of what we were in store for. I hope to make it better for you and your family. I have included this chapter for those who want a true glimpse into our lives on the ketogenic diet. I have separated it into two sections. The first passages reflect days during our first year on the diet; the following passages come from the second year.

It does get easier!

First Year of the Ketogeinc Diet

Monday, October 27, 2003

The challenge of the day: bacon. Well, not actually bacon but "side pork." Not to be confused with salt pork (as one local butcher did). I'm learning a lot about meats and processed foods. Bacon is processed: it starts off as side pork then is smoked and cured. Bryce has had a few seizures on his diet, which we think is from too frequently getting processed foods; thus we must buy side pork rather than bacon.

Bryce wanted bacon for lunch. The two local grocery stores, Shop 'N Save and Giant Eagle, both were fresh out of side pork (or maybe they never carried it, which is especially likely because the one butcher thought it was the same as salt pork). I called a local meat market, Hanson's, last week and placed a special order. Apparently the worker who took my order never passed it on to the store owner, and when we showed up to get it, there was no side pork cut. I was mad and Bryce was upset; he didn't want to eat lunch. I bribed him that if he ate his hamburger (ground beef) and corn for lunch, he'd get "bacon" for dinner. My husband Jeff came through and picked up the side pork on the way home from work. Bryce enjoyed his dinner of bacon and "apple pie" (about one-eighth of a small apple smothered in butter with a pinch of cinnamon, all heated in the microwave oven).

I enjoyed my bacon and apple pie dinner, too. As much as possible I try to eat the same thing as Bryce. Larger amounts with less butter, albeit. I've read in "The Book" (*The Ketogenic Diet; A Treatment for Epilepsy* by Freeman, et al.) that some families eat pizza and breads, etc., in front of their keto-kids. I'm not really sure how this is possible. My husband and I can't do it. I guess we did eat eggplant parmesan with pasta (spaghetti noodles). Bryce had his with long thin strips of zucchini serving as his noodles; he loved it and never asked for ours. So I guess I should clarify: we can't eat something in front of Bryce that Bryce can't have at all. We haven't been able to come to terms with taking Bryce to a restaurant, either, although "The Book" recommends doing it. There's nothing at a restaurant Bryce can eat! "The Book" says we should take Bryce's meal in a Tupperware container and have the restaurant heat it and serve it to him on their dishes.... Could Bryce really be satisfied with chicken and green beans rather than the grilled cheese or chicken nuggets that he previously loved? Perhaps someday we'll get there, but not today. Probably not for awhile. Shortly after Bryce started his "magic diet," as we call it (we got the idea from "The Book"), he asked to go to a restaurant. When I explained we could go, but he'd still have to eat his magic food, he responded "Oh, I don't want to go to a restaurant then." Poor little guy!

◈ *Friday, November 14, 2003*

The food is EVERYWHERE! I took Bryce to a story time at the library last night. It snowed (finally) and I needed to fill up my gas tank before we went home for the night. The service station in town that actually has "service" was closed at 8 pm (what a small town we live in!) I had to go to a self-serve station. As luck would have it, my debit card wouldn't work at the pump. I had to go in; I had to take Bryce. Every blessed inch of that gas station shop was plastered with non-magic-diet-food! Donuts, cookies, candy, juice, even bread! Bryce stared at the bread, mouth gaping, eyes wide, and said "that's bread mom...." Then "is that..." I cut him off "no honey, I'm sorry, it's not on your magic diet." I scooped him up and promptly carried him out of there! My poor boy! He never wined or complained. He's a rock, a pillar of strength! Again, I reminded Bryce and myself that we would not have been there it not been for his magic diet; Bryce was too sick to go to a story time before his diet. And so again I realize how lucky we are!

◈ *Wednesday, November 19, 2003*

Ironically, today is the two-month anniversary of Bryce's first seizure-free day, and also the first day he really complained about being on his magic diet. We just came home from pre-school (his second time back since his seizures progressed) and he told me he didn't want to be on his magic diet anymore; he wanted it to be over. I told him "no," of course, and tried to explain that if he eats things he's not supposed to eat, he'll start having seizures again. Then in the afternoon, he begged for "just one bite" of cheese while I was making his Magic Macaroni and Cheese (with zucchini as noodles) for dinner. Bryce asked me at least ten times, until I finally made him leave the kitchen. He later ate his dinner and snack without any complaints. I hope his negativity was just because he was tired. I know he "gets it" overall. He knows that I picked him up before lunch at daycare so he wouldn't be upset by seeing the other kids eat their regular, non-magic food. Two months down and twenty-two to go!

Thursday, January 1, 2004

Bryce's friend had a party at Chuck E. Cheese. It went great! His mom knows about Bryce's diet and did a good job with putting the pizza in boxes and throwing away the cake as soon as the kids were done. Bryce had a magic pizza and an extra ½ piece of cheesecake, which is always a hit. He never once complained. He really showed a lot of independence by playing the games himself and going through the tunnels with his friends without me frantically hovering over him.

I did get a good understanding of what Bryce means by "the smells" bothering him. We went out to dinner and a party in Meadville for New Year's Eve. Jeff's mother watched the kids. We had to get up at 7 am to make it back for Taylor's birthday party at 11 am. I ate some ham and cheese for breakfast, and didn't eat again until we got back from the party at 2:30 pm. The smell of the pizza was intoxicating! The birthday cake looked divine!

I didn't partake, of course, because Bryce couldn't. I'd recommend these little "exercises" to any keto-mom; it's a humbling lesson about what Bryce faces daily. I'll say it again—he's stronger than me!

Monday, January 5, 2004

Last night I slept without Bryce's baby monitor.... That's monumental! There was a point about six months ago when we slept with Bryce because we were afraid that when he'd seize (as he regularly did in the early morning hours), he'd suffocate and die. It was awful. A couple of times in the last few months I've forgotten to turn the monitor on, but did plug it in during the middle of the night when I remembered. Last night I was able to let it go. How lucky I am!

Tuesday, January 6, 2004

Bryce's grandparents bought him a huge play kitchen for Christmas. We've been struggling with the decision of whether or not to let him have it. We can't decide if it will help him cope, or if the kitchen will make things worse by being yet one more reminder of the food he can't have. I called a children's psychiatry resident at the hospital, and he couldn't decide what would be best, so we've kept it from him so far. Today we changed our minds, however, and gave Bryce the play kitchen. It all started by him seeing a large box in our minivan and remembering the kitchen. He kept asking about it. We told him we weren't sure if he could have it or not. After several "whys" I explained that we don't know if it will make him hungry. He pleaded "It won't; plastic food doesn't smell and only the smells make my belly hungry. I promise I won't eat it." I finally got in touch with the "psychodynamic" specialist psychiatrist (the psychiatry resident referred me), who felt that the kitchen was a great idea. What he said next was even deeper than I, queen of contemplation and deep thought, ever imagined. "Bryce needs to mourn for the food he's missing. The loss of cookies, cakes, chips, breads, candy, etc., is a significant and legitimate loss that must be worked through. It's better to work through those issues now before he starts school, when he'll also have to deal with peer pressures and all the issues that being different brings." It makes sense to me and to Jeff, so we gave Bryce the kitchen. He loves it! We didn't remove any of the non-magic food on advice of the psychiatrist. At one point, I asked for a "magic cookie" as we played. Bryce's response? "We don't have those; you have ice cream!" Bryce also made sure to inform me that his kitchen didn't make him hungry.

  ❦ *Friday, January 16, 2004*

Bryce spent his first half-day at preschool today. He's been going for a few months, but I timed it so it would be after the morning snack but before lunch. Today he ate his breakfast (magic waffle and milk) when his classmates ate their morning snack (cereal and milk). I stayed until the meal was over. He did great. His teachers seemed apprehensive but did pay close attention to the need for him to eat "every last drop." At first they told Bryce he had to stay at the table until everyone was finished, but once I explained how this bothers him they let him go play. The other kids could eat as much as they wanted; Daniel had two bowls of cereal. But when Bryce's waffle is gone, that's it. No more; too bad. He was so excited to get to go to preschool today. I had set his clothes out last night, and he had his sweater, turtleneck, jeans, and socks on, plus was holding his boots and tennis shoes when he first walked out of his bedroom. "I'm ready" he announced; how sweet! Normally it's a chore to get him dressed at all, and he whines that he can't do it himself.

Tuesday, January 20, 2004

"There's nothing like the great outdoors." This was Bryce's remark as we got in the minivan after sled riding at Buhl Park tonight. He was a maniac—fearless and free, flying down the hill with arms over head. As I watched him go down the hill, I was reminded of how lucky we are that he's seizure-free on the keto-genic diet! We had warm tea after our adventure, different than the hot chocolate we used to have, but still okay.

Bryce has been hungry a lot lately. He's also gaining weight—now 34 pounds. He started the diet at 31–32 pounds. Now he's the same weight he was before his epilepsy. He's starting to transition out of an afternoon nap, which gives him more time to be hungry in the afternoon; that stinks.

At church this Sunday, Bryce played with another little boy by crushing real Goldfish Crackers in the mouth of a dinosaur toy. The little boy was eating them but Bryce didn't take a crumb. Bryce's snack was one magic cookie that was gone in one bite. I know he was hungry then, too. He's amazing!

Thursday, January 22, 2004

Bryce asked today if he could have purple dinosaur ice cream with sprinkles after his magic diet is over. That was his favorite flavor at our local ice cream shop. It breaks my heart! So I made magic butterscotch ice cream tonight with dinner. He really seemed to enjoy it. Sometime back in December, he told us he wanted Honeycomb Cereal for Christmas. (The one present we couldn't give him, or should I say the one food of many that he can't have). I've made a habit to ask Bryce regularly if he's hungry or full. I do it so I have a sense of which meals are more or less filling and which times of the day are the worst for him. One time last week when I asked, he said he was full. It was a small meal, I think grilled cheese sandwich, so I didn't believe him. I asked if he was really full, or if he just wanted to make me happy. "I just want to make you happy, mama," he replied. I hate that he's hungry. There was a recent study out of John's Hopkins that looked at six kids on the Atkins diet rather than the ketogenic diet for seizures—how wonderful that would be—no need for hunger (with the Atkins diet, you can eat as much protein and fat as you want). Five out of six kids did well, so further studies will be done. I hope they're in time for Bryce.

⊘ Saturday, January 24, 2004

We went to Pittsburgh to see *The Lion King* last night. My mom bought tickets for Bryce and I as well as my sister and her two kids. It was spectacular! Bryce was enthralled for the entire 2½-hour performance. I realize the tickets were expensive and it was very nice of her to take us. But my mother made me very angry tonight. She ate through the entire performance! I couldn't believe it; there was constant wrapper crinkling! Food is not allowed in the theater AND her grandson can't eat extra snacks! People, even family, just don't get it! Luckily, Bryce and I sat in front of my mother and sister and I really don't think he knew what was going on. But I did! At one point, my mom asked if she should have brought milk for Bryce to have at her house. "No, mom, it's cream...heavy whipping cream! And I have to measure it. And, he can't have as much as he wants!" I'm a little frustrated about the hunger and the restriction and the ignorance of others!

⊘ Sunday, January 25, 2004

I just watched *First Do No Harm* starring Meryl Streep. Wow! It took me about ten months to muster the emotional strength to watch it. Jeff started to watch it with me but had to leave the room. I can't explain why I felt the need to watch it, but I'm glad I did. It's renewed for me the feeling of how lucky and blessed we are that we're on the ketogenic diet, that it's working, that we really only had 2½ awful months of seizures, that our doctors were for the diet, and that I have my son back! I didn't buy the movie; a patient of mine, Becky, knows about Bryce and purchased it for me. She had to search online for it because it's not at any of the video stores. That in itself was touching. The movie was produced by Jim Abrams, who has a son Charlie who was on the diet for over six years. Now Charlie is off the diet and medication- and seizure-free. Some of the actors in the movie had been previously on the ketogenic diet. At the end they showed them along with a statement of how long each person was on the diet (generally 3–6 years) and how long they've been seizure-free (25–50 years). How incredible to see a normal older adult with a caption "Joe Blow was on the ketogenic diet from 1960 to 1963.... He has been seizure-free for 27 years." I feel like I've been frustrated with the diet for the past two weeks, almost engaging in self-pity for Bryce having to be on it. Now I'm reminded how foolish it is to think that way! We are so, so, so very lucky to be on the ketogenic diet! One of my favorite scenes in the movie was at the end. Robbie (the keto-kid) was being blessed by a priest who quoted Matthew 17, which talked about Jesus healing a boy with epilepsy. His disciples asked how He did it, since they tried to heal the boy and couldn't. His response: "prayer and fasting."

Tuesday, January 27, 2004

We went to Pittsburgh for Bryce's check-up with Dr. Williams today. The weather was awful, but we plugged through it. We wouldn't miss the appointment for anything! It was great— she's letting us decrease Bryce's Depakote to two pills twice a day instead of two and a half in the morning and two in the evening. She wants to keep Bryce on the Depakote for a year, then we'll wean off and hopefully he'll be med-free and seizure-free. Bryce had to have labs drawn again; poor guy!

Thursday, January 29, 2004

Bryce gave me the ultimate compliment today. I made a new recipe at his request—a magic peanut butter sandwich (really macadamia nut butter) with blueberries as the jelly. Also, I threw in a butterscotch butter ball for dessert (butter rolled in a ball, dipped in water with a few drops of butterscotch flavoring and sweetener). Bryce ate his lunch, said "that was yummy," then asked if he could still have a magic peanut butter and blueberry sandwich and a butterscotch ball after his magic diet is over! WOW!

I spent eight to nine hours cooking today—3 meals plus fifteen waffles and 5 cheesecakes—a grand total of 23 meals. The fact that Bryce likes the food and that it makes the diet a little easier, makes it all worthwhile.

Monday, May 24, 2004

We went on our first big weekend trip to visit our friends Nicole, Alan, and Maddy. I tackled it all myself: two kids, scale, recipe book, lots of keto-foods, and myself. We bought a cooler that plugs into the car, which helped. Bryce and I agreed on a meal plan ahead of time, and I made him sign it as usual. On Friday, we all went to Kings Island. I made blue-colored frozen whipped cream with chocolate flavoring, blueberries on the bottom, and nut sprinkles for his snack. The first aid office kept it in the freezer for us. We all had peanut butter and jelly sandwiches (magic macadamia nut butter and sliced blueberries for Bryce). I learned that the park snow cone machines, unlike home snow cone machines, use ice only (not sugar and salt); I was able to give him a huge snow cone dripping with his magic Kool-Aid. He was in heaven!

On Sunday, Maddy (5-years-old) had her birthday party at a dude ranch. I was so proud of myself for simulating the party meal (fruit, veggies, and cupcakes) with a chocolate magic cupcake, carrots dipped in macadamia nut butter, a few strawberry slices, and a few watermelon slices. Little did I know the day included a marshmallow roast! Crap! My perfect keto-simulation ruined! At one point we were on a hayride before the marshmallow roast, and an excited little girl was asking her mom when we'd have the marshmallow roast and if she could eat them. Sarcastically, her mom replied "No, you can't eat them. You can look at them, touch them, smell them, and cook them, then you have to give them away...." Welcome to our world, I thought! But give them away is exactly what Bryce did. He insisted on roasting three marshmallows and having me eat them. He even made me lick the stick clean each time (my great little keto-scraper!). He did amazingly well! I gave him a carrot from his lunch after each marshmallow, so at least he had something to eat (lunch was immediately following the roast). He really liked the roasting part, and asked to do it again at our cottage at Chautauqua Lake in June. He was really excited when I told him we can have a magic hot dog roast!

Wednesday, June 16, 2004

Tonight, I made a huge batch of 12 muffins, and I colored then green and called them "Shrek Muffins." The movie *Shrek II* just came out and we saw it last weekend. They were a huge hit; I think he's eaten 6 of the 12 already. And what an easy meal for me—just heat in the microwave or toaster oven and serve. No counting or measuring required (it was all done ahead of time).

Second Year of the Ketogenic Diet

Monday, September 20, 2004

Last Friday, Bryce's teacher gave all the kids a balloon and a Tootsie Pop sucker to celebrate their first full week of kindergarten. She forewarned me, and I packed him a butter sucker to have in place of the Tootsie Pop. I was shocked when I came home from work on Friday to find a Tootsie Pop on the dining room table! I was mad that my instructions weren't followed… mad that Bryce carried forbidden candy. He asked to trade it in for YuGiOh cards; I decided to allow the trade, praising him for leaving the candy out for me and for not eating it. I found out by talking to the teacher today that Bryce didn't want the butter sucker and he convinced the teacher he'd take home the Tootsie Pop to trade. What a little rascal! I did make an on-the-spot decision and asked the teacher to make Bryce trade for a prize at school rather than carry candy home. I don't want to risk temptation.

Monday, November 1, 2004

For the first time in a year, I was able to enjoy myself at a kids' play land. Gracie was asleep and I was chit-chatting with another mom at McDonald's play land; Bryce was busy crawling and sliding through all the "rat mazes." I actually didn't worry he would seize inside one of those tubes when I lost sight of him. It was so relieving! I'm not walking on eggshells at home anymore either; I don't worry Bryce is seizing when he doesn't answer me immediately or when he's playing in another room. My husband

Jeff says he hasn't worried about Bryce in months…I'm jealous! Better late than never.

Wednesday, November 3, 2004

Bryce said something today that warmed my heart. We were in the car after school, talking about his day. He said "Mommy, I don't ever want to cheat on my magic diet; I'm having too much fun." Too much fun in school, I questioned? "No, fun all the time." What a magical little being!

Thursday, November 4, 2004

I was called by the school nurse today and amazingly my first thought was not "Oh my, Bryce had a seizure." The problem was an itchy butt—to the point that Bryce was crying about it. Poor little fellow! He knew enough (of hemorrhoids) to tell the teacher he needed to go to the nurse, call his mom, and get some cream. A 5-year-old shouldn't know about Preparation H! But, I'll take the hemorrhoids rather than the seizures any day. It's all worth it!

Saturday, November 6, 2004

Today was a milestone. Bryce took a friend from kindergarten to the movies. I explained the diet to Hayden's mom before we went, so she packed pretzels as a treat for Hayden and I brought macadamia nuts for Bryce and bottled water for both. Hayden finished his water and wanted a pop—it was fine since Bryce doesn't like pop. The day was a great success! We watched *The Incredibles*. It was a joy to see Bryce hoot and holler with his little friend. And the popcorn smell didn't seem as bad as before—I guess this too gets better with time.

ᴄᴋ Wednesday, January 12, 2005

After all this time on the diet, it's easy to fall into a false sense of security, a sort of complacency. Yesterday, while I was fixing dinner, I gave Gracie a cracker to eat in her highchair to keep her occupied. I've been giving her Gerber crackers and veggie puffs, as well as Kix cereal for weeks now, and Bryce hasn't seemed to mind. Yesterday he did. He asked if Grace was eating a "big cracker that's not on my magic diet." Yes, I responded, and asked if it bothered him. He said it did, because it was one big piece. It was about two inches in diameter. I quickly broke it up into about six pieces, and this seemed to help Bryce. Lately he's asked for things to be in "one big piece," I suppose out of frustration that all of his food is chopped up into little pieces and spread around on the plate to make it look like more! After our exchange, I launched into a discussion about non-magic diet foods. I explained that mommy gives up some foods that aren't on Bryce's diet, like cookies and cakes and candy. Grace has never had one piece of candy, and Bryce had lots of candy by the time he was one (before his magic diet). Grace is just a baby, however, and she must eat lots of different foods including crackers in order to stay healthy; we all have different diets. Bryce seemed to be satisfied with this. Just to be safe, though, I'll cut up Grace's cracker next time.

ᴄᴋ Tuesday, January 18, 2005

Bryce had his first playdate WITHOUT me today. It was with one of his friends from kindergarten, Sergio. Sergio's mom picked Bryce up from school and he stayed at their house until Jeff got home from work (about 2 hours). I talked with Sergio's mom last night, and made sure to stress the "nothing to eat or drink but water" rule, except for the snack I sent with him (two mini-strawberry/blueberry muffins and butter) and Crystal Light Raspberry Lemonade mix (I sent one canister of mix and asked her to make it). They had a ball and there were no diet misadventures. I guess I'm finally cutting the umbilical cord. I'm sure it didn't hurt that I talked with Bryce multiple times about saying "no, thank you, that's not on my magic diet" if offered a snack other than his own, or that I threatened him with "no more playdates" if he cheated at Sergio's house. Bryce is an amazing little boy!

Saturday, February 19, 2005

Today was a milestone. I took Bryce to a restaurant for the first time since being on his diet. We're trying to sell our house (never a dull moment here) and so while we were having a showing, I took the kids and my girlfriend and we went shopping. We started the afternoon by going to Subway. We took bacon, carrots, and cream for Bryce and had it heated up there. He asked for a Subway bowl, so we transferred his bacon into it. My girlfriend Heidi and I had salads (no croutons, of course; they bother Bryce). He did great! To my surprise, he was really excited to even be at the restaurant in the first place. He certainly noticed the non-magic food. We were playing "I spy" and he spied "something round and yummy with chocolate chips." Also "something brown and fluffy and you eat it on a sandwich." Bless his little heart!

Thursday, March 3, 2005

Yesterday Bryce's grandparents came up for dinner and took Bryce to a toy store to pick his birthday present. We had salmon; he had crab legs. The family dinners are becoming less and less of a big deal. This time we served the food "family style" whereas we usually make our plates in the kitchen and bring them into the dining room. Bryce's other grandparents came tonight for cheesecake; magic for Bryce and regular for us. Again, it went off without a hitch.

Saturday, April 2, 2005

I've been in contact with another keto-mom; unfortunately her little 3½-year-old little Chloe isn't doing very well on the diet. She isn't old enough to understand that you can't hurl keto-food across the room or take a few bites then spit it out. I feel so badly for them; I wish the diet would be as helpful for Chloe as it has been for Bryce. I've been sharing recipes with her mom, and trying to help as much as I can. Bryce and I added Chloe to his nightly prayers. When I explained to Bryce that I was trying to help Chloe's mom with her magic diet, he listened carefully then asked, "You mean you want the magic diet to help Chloe so that she can have a wonderful life like me?" Wow!

Wednesday, April 6, 2005

I was called by the school nurse again today because Bryce threw up at lunch. It was the third time in a month and about the fifth or sixth time overall. At first I thought it was mixing oil in milk that caused the vomiting; now I think it's simply the high-fat meal. This time, Bryce apparently complained that there were "black things" in his hot dog and corn. It was pepper, which he usually likes in his corn (along with salt). The thought of it must have gagged him or something, but I'm told the end result was that he yakked in his food, again. I went to the school and let Bryce come outside with me for a few minutes (it was an unseasonably beautiful 78 degree day). I gave him half of a chocolate cupcake to eat; I figured I'd get some fat back into him, assuming he probably threw up the butter. He was still in 3+ (high) ketosis tonight, so it must have worked.

Jeff and I both had the same thought on the matter—if this is the least of our problems with this diet, we're doing fine. I immediately thought of poor little Chloe; she's been hospitalized several times for acidosis because of the ketogenic diet. Some kids get kidney stones or pancreatitis or recurrent infections from immunodeficiency. As tempting as it is to lament in self-pity, just a little, I must remember how lucky we are!

Sunday, June 19, 2005

The past month and a half has been an emotional roller-coaster. So much has happened; I almost don't know where to begin.

Bryce graduated from kindergarten. It was an especially sweet victory for Jeff and me, given that when his seizures were at their worst, the prognosis was grim. It was a joy to see him in his little white graduation cap. We had a meeting at his school, and although the consensus was that he could proceed to first grade, Jeff and I ultimately decided to keep him back in kindergarten another year to mature. I was nervous to tell Bryce about our decision. I explained that not all kids have to go to first grade, and that some kids would rather stay in kindergarten where there is more time to play. I stressed to Bryce that he is very smart, but that we just didn't think he'd like all of the extra work in first grade. He thought for a minute then paraphrased: "You mean because I'm so smart, you're rewarding me by letting me stay in kindergarten another year? Yeah!" Next, I reminded him that he'd no longer be the smallest kid in the class. That was met with an even bigger "yeah!" I feel very good about our decision.

Bryce had his overnight EEG on June 1st. It was the best experience we've had of the four. The tech placed the leads on

Bryce in his room, which was wonderful since Bryce could watch TV during it (a great distraction) and I could lay in bed with him (for one great big reassuring hug). At the conclusion, the tech even leaked that there was "nothing major." I was flying high for a week after that. My daydreaming of diet-free days increased exponentially; I began to create a mental list of guests for our "no more diet" picnic.

About a week after the EEG, I called the nurse practioner and asked for the results. To my great disappointment and surprise, they were NOT NORMAL!! During the 10-hour test, there was one brief episode of spike and wave on the EEG, although Bryce didn't clinically have any seizures. I had so many questions.... If we would stay on the diet longer, would there be less chance of seizing again? (She didn't know). What if the diet doesn't work the second time? (There's always that chance, she said). What would you do if it were your son? (She couldn't answer).

The doctor didn't call me for a week. I later found that she was on vacation; it would have been nice to have been informed. In desperation, I called several other doctors who would give me the courtesy of their time. The best advice came from not only a pediatric neurologist, but THE pediatric neurologist regarding the ketogenic diet. Dr. John Freeman was very kind to take my call. When I began rambling about how thankful I was that he'd talk to me and how I knew that his time was valuable and I'd be brief and I started into the 60 second summary of the past two years, he interrupted me, "Slow down, slow down." What an amazing, kind soul! Dr. Freeman felt that a brief spike and wave may or may not be significant. He felt that the only way to know was to wean off the diet. He gave me advice on a newer way to wean. When I asked him what the chances were that the diet wouldn't work a second time, he quickly extinguished my fears with a confident, "It will." I asked him when I could feel comfortable that he wouldn't seize. "When you're 72," he teased."

Very true! He actually felt that if Bryce doesn't seize within one month after cessation of the diet, it would be a pretty good sign. I LITERALLY felt a ton of bricks being lifted from my shoulders after we talked.

In my analytical, mathematically thinking, ketogenic-calculating mind, I've computed that Bryce only had a less than one second abnormality out of the 36,000 seconds during his 10-hour EEG. Jeff brought up the point that perhaps a certain percentage of the population would have bursts of spikes and waves on an extended EEG, if we tested them. I will continue to pray myself and to ask for prayers; at this point that's all I can do.

🌊 *Tuesday, July 12, 2005*

The day has finally come. Tonight, after work, Jeff and I had a family meeting with Bryce. We announced that his diet is OVER! We celebrated by going to Eat N' Park; Bryce's grandparents and aunt Darci met us there. Bryce ordered a cheeseburger and fries; he ate every last fry and most of the cheeseburger. Although completely stuffed, he even managed to pack away a whole smiley face cookie! It was glorious! I cried, of course, but just a little. After dinner, Jeff and I took Bryce to the grocery store. We just hung back and let him "buy" whatever he wanted. It was interesting to see his choices—bananas and apples, then a Lunchables meal, then Trix yogurt and Lucky Charms cereal and Pop-Tarts. He completely passed the cookie and donut section, but did "order" a Panera asiago cheese bagel for breakfast.

There are so many emotions, one after the other and then back again. Immediately, I felt elation, then relief and gratitude and anxiety. I felt freedom and awe; awe that we've been given such a miracle as the ketogenic diet.

Friday, August 12, 2005

It's been exactly one month, and he's still seizure-free. THIS IS A TRUE MODERN DAY MIRACLE. I am so, so, so very thankful to God! And to all of the neurologists who have worked to develop and promote the ketogenic diet. And to all of the children and parents who have come before us. It's simply overwhelming. It's simply wonderful!

I can honestly say that every bit of every sacrifice was worth it. I would do it all over again in a heartbeat. I thank God every day for the ketogenic diet, still. I hope I never forget how lucky we are.

That hope leads me to my final thought. I wish ALL children would become seizure-free on the ketogenic diet. I don't know why Bryce was so lucky when other children, like Chloe, are not. Jeff and I have wrestled with that question on many occasions. We are no more deserving of a miracle than anyone else, and yet it has been given to us. Bryce has been blessed; our family has been blessed. And so I will end this beautiful story with my favorite prayer "Thank You, God, for the ketogenic diet and for making Bryce seizure-free."

APPENDIX

A. Halloween Note

Dear Neighbor,

We are asking for your help again this year with Trick-or-Treat for our son Bryce. He is on a special diet to control his seizures. The diet is very strict and he can't have any chips, cookies, candy, etc. Of course, this makes Halloween a little challenging. Please give Bryce this treat when we come around on Friday evening for Trick-or-Treat. It will really help him enjoy the holiday despite his restrictions.

Bryce is 5-years-old and will be wearing a purple Yu-Gi-Oh outfit; I've enclosed a picture to help you recognize him.

If you are not planning on participating in Trick-or-Treat, please jot down your street address on this note and drop it in our mail slot so that we may give it to another address.

Thank you in advance for your help!

Jeff and Debbie Snyder

B. Note to School Lunch Moms

To: School Lunch Moms
Re: Bryce Snyder

I would greatly appreciate your help with my son, Bryce, at lunchtime. He has epilepsy and is on a special diet called the ketogenic diet. We call it his "magic diet" because it makes his seizures "disappear." He has been on it for almost two years, and we've been blessed that he has been seizure-free for that time. The diet is very high in fat and calories are strictly limited (he only gets 75% of calories for his age, and 90% of those calories are from fat). I must calculate a recipe for every meal (with exact protein, fat, and carb amounts) and then weigh it exactly on a gram scale. Therefore, other than the items I send, Bryce cannot share food with other children and cannot have anything to eat or drink except water. Please realize that this includes sugar-free and calorie-free drinks; often drinks that say sugar-free actually have sugar in them and can cause Bryce to have a seizure.

I try very hard to make foods similar to "kid foods" that Bryce used to eat, and that he sees other kids eat. This helps him feel included and to stick to his diet.

The diet doesn't work if he doesn't get it all, especially if he doesn't get all of the oil and butter. If a piece of food falls on the floor, it is to be picked up, wiped off and eaten. In the case of a major spill or other major problem, please call me.

If there will be some special occasion and I know ahead of time, I can usually make something for Bryce that will allow him to feel included; I would greatly appreciate a phone call (no matter how short the notice) regarding any special treats. Thanks so much!

C. Note to Kindergarten Teacher and School Nurse

Re: Bryce Snyder

A. Food

Mrs. Povanda,

Bryce is on the ketogenic diet to control his seizures. We call it his "magic diet" because it makes his seizures "disappear." He had been on it for one year, and we are blessed that he has been seizure-free for almost one year. I have enclosed several handouts for your information. The diet is very strict and limited in calories. I must calculate a recipe for every meal and then weight it exactly on a gram scale. Thus, Bryce can not have anything to eat or drink other than water (in addition to what I send). Even some drinks (and suntan lotions, toothpastes, etc.) that say they are sugar-free actually have sugar in them and can cause Bryce to have a seizure.

Unfortunately, the world we live in centers around food. This is one of the greatest challenges for Bryce and our family. He does take ownership in his diet, and understands that if he cheats, he may have a seizure. I am hopeful he'll do well in kindergarten with those issues. I have become very creative and can reproduce many kid-type foods like magic pizza, magic waffles, magic muffins, magic cupcakes, magic cheesecake, etc. If there will be some special occasion and I know ahead of time, I can usually make something for Bryce that will allow him to feel included.

Please feel free to tell his classmates, if needed, about his magic diet. (In his previous preschool, the teachers weren't permitted to discuss any health issues without the parent's permission; you have my permission). We are very open and forthright about Bryce's seizures and his diet. This may be needed, if you notice other children offering Bryce their food, as an example.

Bryce really is doing well and, thank God, is just like any other normal kid now. He needs help to "scrape" his bowls/plates when he's finished, because the diet is very exact and only works if he gets every last drop. That's about all the special attention he needs, however, and otherwise will be just one of the class.

Please feel free to call me at work (xxx-xxxx) or at home (xxx-xxxx) if you have any questions at any time.

Thank you! We look forward to a wonderful year!

Mrs. Debbie Snyder

cc: School nurse

B. Seizures

Two years ago, Bryce had three different types of seizures: tonic (jerking/stiff/grandmal kind), myoclonic jerks (he'd fall back on his head as if someone pushed him) and atypical absence (his eyes would flicker, his hand would tremble, and he couldn't talk). He hasn't had a seizure for almost two years. He previously would smell a fruity smell (that wasn't there) prior to a seizure, or everything would look red. If he tells you he smells or sees this, lay him down safely and call me, please.

I have enclosed instructions for seizure care. If Bryce has a seizure, please

1. note the time on your watch
2. turn him on his side; NOTHING IN HIS MOUTH
3. remove objects that are nearby that he can hit into
4. call me; I'll come immediately
5. you may certainly call 911 if that is your policy—tell the squad: no sugar in the IV!!
6. if a seizure lasts more than 4 or 5 minutes, administer Diastat rectally (there are instruction in the medicine case).

THANK YOU for your help! Please feel free to call me at work M,T, F (xxx-xxxx) or at home W, Th (xxx-xxxx), or page me (xxx-xxxx) if you have any questions at any time.

Thank you.

Debbie Snyder

Grandma's Instructions for a Parents' Weekend Away

BRYCE'S FOOD INSTRUCTIONS

Bryce decided to eat the same meals for Friday, Saturday, and Sunday. This should help to make it easier for you.

Breakfast: Blueberry Waffle

1. The waffle is in the freezer in a freezer bag marked "weekend." Toast the waffle in the toaster oven for 4-5 minutes, then melt the butter on it by spreading it around (the butter is already measured and on the plate with the waffle in the freezer).
2. Measure 10 grams of cream in a small plastic cup (it's okay if it's 10.5-11 grams) then add these:
   i. 2 depakote sprinkle capsules (pour in the sprinkles)
   ii. carnitore tablet, crushed
   iii. 1 tablespoon (roughly) of Cal-Mag-Zinc (in the refrigerator door)
   iv. 10-15 drops of liquid sweetener
   v. enough water to fill up half of the cup

3. Put a straw cut to 2/3 the original size in the cream. Make sure he gets every last drop of milk and scrape the plate from the waffle with a spatula when he's done.

Lunch: Macaroni and Cheese

1. Take from freezer, remove foil covering, and cover with plastic wrap instead. Heat in microwave 1 minute. If the center is still frozen, heat another 30 seconds. It may be too hot to eat when its done; you can put it back in the freezer for a minute to get it cool enough to eat.
2. Serve with keto-Kool-Aid or lemonade. Only two glasses of lemonade per day.
3. Give him his Looney Tunes vitamin to chew if he didn't ask for it at breakfast.
4. Help him spoon up the butter at the end, then scrape the bowl with a spatula to get it all.

Dinner: Hot Dog and Apple Pie

1. Heat the square container in the microwave for 1 minute (crack the lid first).
2. Measure 10 grams of cream (10.5-11 grams is okay). Add to cream:
   a. 10-15 drops of liquid sweetener
   b. one carnitore tablet crushed
   c. enough water to fill the plastic cup ½ way
   d. if he wants chocolate or strawberry milk, you can add a pinch of chocolate pudding mix or strawberry Jell-O mix.
3. Help him get every last drop of milk and scrape the container with a spatula. He can have a few ounces of Kool-Aid ("juice") after he drinks his milk.

Snack: Blueberry Ice Cream

1. They are in the door of the freezer. They get really hard, so thaw them on the counter for 20 minutes or so before you're ready to serve, or, if you forget, defrost in the microwave for 20 seconds.
2. His Depakote and a carnitore are already in the ice cream.
3. He can have a few ounces of Kool-Aid ("juice") after he finishes his ice cream.

INDEX

Bacon (*continued*)
  hard boiled eggs and, 50
  ice cream and, 72
  quiche, 64
  turkey and, with cheese and milk, 95
  yogurt swirl and, 66–67
bananas and eggs, 56
bartering and negotiating meals, 22
beans, green
  bacon and, 71–72
  bacon and, with carrots, 68
  bottom round roast with, 79–80
  burger and hot dog with, 78, 89
  burger and, 76–78
  hot dog and mashed potato with, 90
  snow crab and, with pudding, 92–93
beef, 73–80
  bottom round roast with green beans, 79–80
  burger and blueberries, 75
  burger with carrots, 74
  burger with cheese, 73–74
  burger, hot dog and green beans, 78, 89
  green beans and, 76–78
  ground (hamburger), fat vs. protein content of, 73
  meatballs and apple pie, 74–75
  spaghetti with meatballs, 98–99
  tacos, 79
  top round roast with apple pie, 80
Bickford flavorings, 32, 35
birthday parties, 24–25, 134, 138–139
blueberries
  burger and, 75
  eggs and, 56–57
  milk and, 106
bologna
  and cheese sandwich, 103–104
  strawberries and, 91–92
bottom round roast with green beans, 79–80
bread, 35, 101. *See also* sandwiches
breakfast meals, 45–65
bulk cooking, 33
Burger King, 22

butter
  apple chips and bacon with, 108
  apple-cinnamon soy crisps and bacon with, 110
  bacon and butter dip, 108
  mini-muffins and, 110

Cal-Mag-Zinc, 36
Calcimix, 36
calcium, 36
calculating meal values, 30–31, 43–44
calories, 10
  flexibility with, 27
  increasing intake of, 26–27
candy, 40, 135
  molds for, 11
carbohydrate values, 32–33, 39
carnitine, 38
Carnitor, 38
carrots
  bacon and, with beans, 68
  bacon and, with muffin, milk, 69–70
  burger with, 74
  chicken nuggets and, 81–83
  macadamia nuts and, 109–110
  smoked sausage and peas with, 91
  turkey and, 93–94
cereals, 40
  Cream of Wheat, 64–65
  low-carb, 63, 63
  milk and, 62
  oatmeal, 65
cheating, xi, 24
cheese, 105
  and bologna sandwich, 103–104
  burger with, 73–74
  cheese puffs and milk, 106
  chicken and, 86
  chicken and, with bacon, 84
  eggplant parmesan, 99–100
  eggs and, with apple juice or strawberries, 57–58
  grilled cheese sandwich, 102
  macaroni and cheese, 97–98
  quiche, 64
  spaghetti squash with, 99

KETOGENIC DIET TITLES

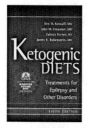
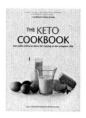
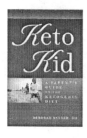
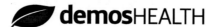